Today Is My Monday. . .

Beginning tips when getting started on your Health and Fitness Journey

Alura T Jefferies
C.P.T. / N.C.

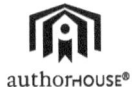

authorHOUSE®

AuthorHouse™
1663 Liberty Drive
Bloomington, IN 47403
www.authorhouse.com
Phone: 1-800-839-8640

Published by AuthorHouse 08/10/2012

ISBN: 978-1-4772-2445-8 (sc)
ISBN: 978-1-4772-2444-1 (e)

Library of Congress Control Number: 2012911049

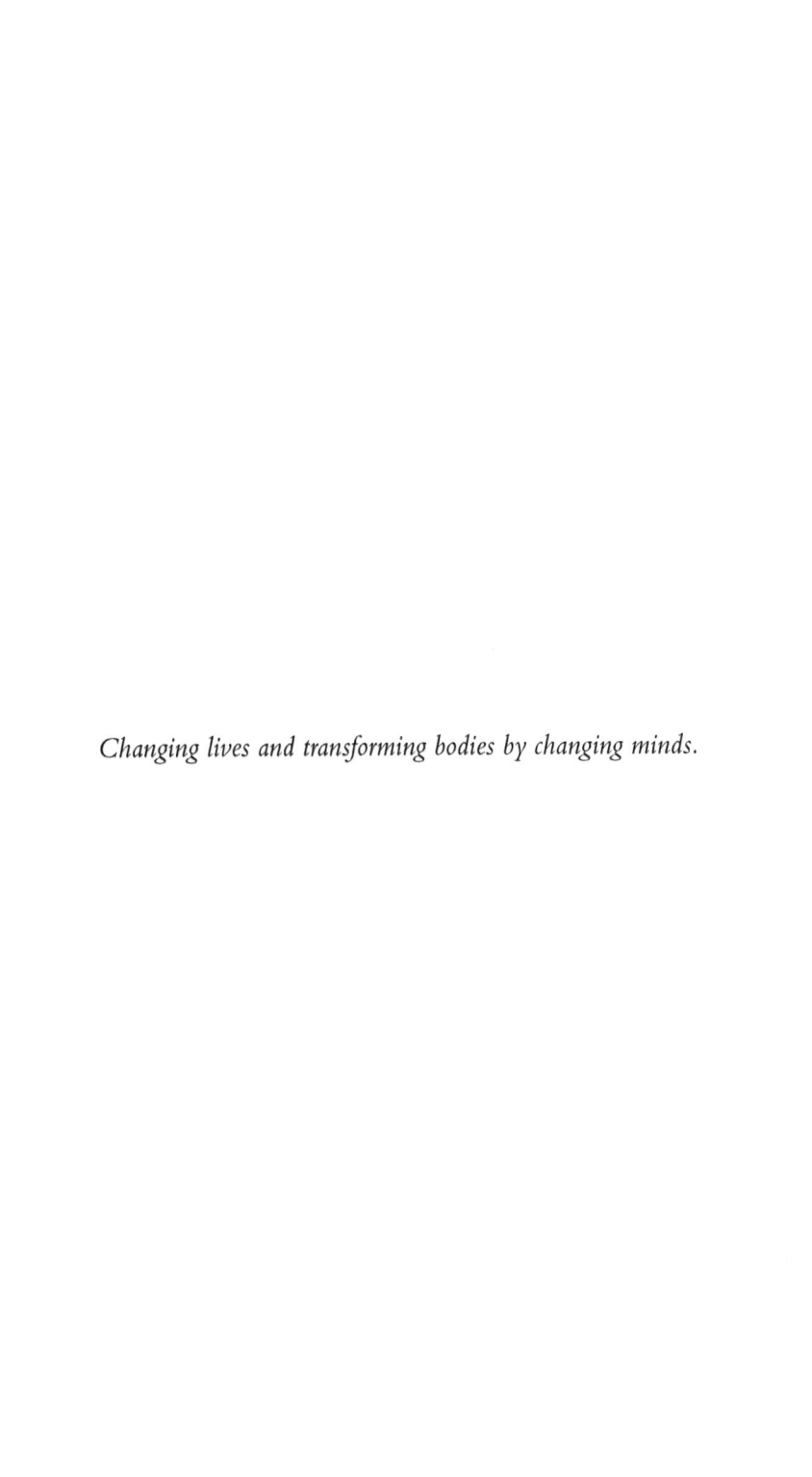

Changing lives and transforming bodies by changing minds.

Contents

Foreword

As a Certified Personal Trainer and Nutrition Consultant, I love health and fitness. I try to keep myself educated and up to date on all things fitness and good health. I do courses and seminars to seek out any information that I can in order to be able to help others. I own and have come across many books that have been written to help and inspire others in their own fitness journeys. There are many that are very helpful and have changed many lives, but in my research there are a lot that read like stereo instructions. To be very truthful and honest, many are hard to read and understand. I thought to myself that if I am having a hard time following and understanding the how and the why as fitness Trainer then imagine the lay person's response. That's the person that has no clue of where to start, what to do or where to go first. Well at least that is what I run across on a daily basis in my profession. People have very busy lives with their jobs and families and need something that is simplified and straight to the point. Getting healthy in the beginning can be difficult and very confusing. Some of the information starts as if the person who is reading already knows exactly what they speak of. In most instances that is not the case. There are tons of people in whom which have no knowledge about where point "A" is when trying to get healthy or how to get there. In this case, I wanted to write a straight to the point, basic fundamental book that will hold your attention as you get you started on your fitness journey.

I started writing this book after my entire life was turned upside down. I was already a Certified Personal Trainer but I was not living up to my potential. At that time I just did enough to look better than the client. I did not practice what I preached so to speak. But after the life that I knew crumbled, I used my misfortune as fuel to my fire and transformed my body into what I always envisioned it to be. I didn't do it because of my situation, but I did it despite of it. It made me feel so much better physically as well as mentally. I think I used my tragedy to finally gain triumph over my body and my bad eating habits that had controlled me for so long. In my very trying time I did not turn to food as my numbing drug of choice as I so often times did, but I wanted to turn to something that was beneficial for me in the long run. I told myself that I had the control and that day was to become forever know as My Monday.

INTRODUCTION ─────────────

Our Bodies are our main asset and as far as I know we only get one of them on this side of the earth. We use many common excuses on why we can't take better care of our bodies. A few of the excuses deal with time, expense, aches and pains, energy and others. The list of excuses is endless. All these excuses can be dispelled always. The fact of the matter is that we are ailing and dying daily because of the excuses. Obesity causes many deaths and preventable diseases. We must get serious about our health or we will be doomed to live a lifeless life or worse be destined to an early death.

In this book I will show you how to gradually begin to change your life one day at a time. My main objective is to get you to take control of your life by understanding food, its purpose and not to be controlled by it. There are countless fly by night, get slim and healthy over night advertisements that build you up to let you down because there is no clarification or long term solution offered to you. It has been my experience when trying to obtain a healthy and fit lifestyle it goes right back to plain ole proper nutrition and exercise. Those two together always work and they never get outdated.

If you read and follow these simple, plain English

steps and gradually incorporate them into your life then you will gain success. Everyone has a starting point which in my opinion is the hardest thing to do. It starts with making a clear decision and continues with focus and determination.

Today is my Monday was written out of my genuine love and concern for people. I hope that it will help you gain some knowledge and understanding that is needed along your fitness journey. So let's get to it. Today is your Monday!

Speak with your Doctor before starting your fitness journey

This is number one because it is very important to set up a Doctor's visit before starting your fitness journey. It is always a great thing to begin to get healthy, but keeping this very important step is crucial to the whole entire process. There are many things that are of vital importance to you that you need to know before you begin. The Doctor will administer several test that the results will play a very important role in where you should begin. At this time you will need to make an appointment for a full physical. The doctor will check out something such as, Lung capacity, blood pressure, blood levels, sugar levels, and bone and joint to name a few.

If there are any specific concerns that you have be sure that you mention it to your Doctor so that he or she might exam it to determine its causes. If there are no issues to concern yourself with the doctor will give the okay to move forward. If there are any issues that demand attention, he or she will give special instructions to you on how and where to begin with your fitness journey. It might be a specified nutrition plan or specific instructions to follow when exercising. Remember not to skip this very critical step. This step is also helpful because it lets you know where you are starting out from. So when you are healthier you can look back and see how far you have come.

SET A DATE

When starting anything that is important to you must set a date. If you are planning a wedding or an important event there is a lot of preparation involved in preparing for this event. I am not saying take six months to prepare to start your fitness journey, but I am saying the moment that you decide in your mind that you are going to start to make an effort to change your life you must plan and set a specific date to start that. The advice that I give is to make the decision, plan a celebration for the departure of your old life and the entrance of your new one, plan a date and then follow through.

Normally I tell my clients to do this over the weekend. I tell them to take that weekend to enjoy all of the terrible foods that they desire. I allow them to stay up late doing whatever activities that they chose. This serves as a going away party for them to try to mentally prepare them for their new lifestyle. After the going away party, most of the times, it is on that Monday it will be time to show and prove. They will have set the date and now it is time to get started. I am not saying that you will be perfect in your new lifestyle but at least you will have set a date and finally followed through with plans to try. I promise you there will be times when you fall of the wagon, but it will be up to you to see the benefits of having good health and that alone will give you the encouragement to start again clean.

KNOW YOUR NUMBERS

Just as it is important to get your numbers from the doctor for your health's sake, it is equally important to know your starting numbers for your sanity's sake. Knowing your starting weight, body fat, blood pressure and measurement might prove to be very difficult to hear in the beginning but it has a very important role for you as you progress. The initial information can sometimes come to be a shock to you but at least you have that information and the good thing is that you are determined to do something about it.

The doctor will most likely let you know your weight, height and blood pressure. With obesity being on the rise most will even be able to tell you your body fat percentage. Body fat percentage is that percentage of body mass that is not made up of bone, muscle, connective tissue and fluids. If your body fat percentage is too high then it becomes of grave importance to lower it. We do that by proper nutrition (taking in less fat) and exercise (burning some of the stored fat that we already have.) Ideally we would like to have the body fat percentage below 30%. Anymore puts us at a greater risk for heart attacks, strokes, diabetes, fertility issues, and certain cancers. Body fat percentage is measured mostly by Fat Calipers and digital machines. It goes off of your height and your weight.

Knowing these numbers and keeping a record of them will later serve a whole other purpose. If you are serious and work hard each time you check this information again you will begin to see your numbers get better and better. I recommend that you have your numbers rechecked every four weeks. If your numbers stay the same as far as the weight on the scale, it is not necessarily a bad thing. This is when it becomes important to keep up with your measurement and the body fat percentage. The scale does not tell the entire story. If you see some changes in things such as the measurements and body fat percentage that will for most people motivate you to want to do more. Accurately keeping track of your numbers will charge you either way it goes. If there is no change, that in itself will hopefully fuel your fire to reevaluate and rededicate yourself to the commitment you've made to yourself.

Grab a book that you have specifically designed for the record keeping process and be consistent with keeping track of your progress. There are books for sale made especially for this purpose or you can make your own out of a tablet or notebook. Not knowing how far we have come has killed a lot of healthy lifestyles. We see ourselves everyday and are not able to see the changes that seem to be insignificant, but if we write it down the numbers will not lie. I promise that doing this will motivate you to keep going because you are able to physically see your progress in black and white. Picture taking is also a great way to track your progress. This can be done every four weeks as well.

Set Realistic Goals

There isn't anything more discouraging to a Personal Trainer than to have a client or a potential client tell you that they would like to lose 50 pounds for a cruise that they are going on in June when it is May already. As a person that understands how the body works and understands why those kinds of request are very unrealistic and unattainable. Not to mention that they are very unhealthy to attempt.

I am not saying have low expectations, but let's face it, you must be realistic. The main reason people quit their workout and nutrition plans is because of the feeling that it did not work. They started out with setting their goals that were not unattainable for the time frame. We tend to set the bar too high and when we don't reach our goals we give up completely. We cannot expect that after many years as a couch potato we magically to turn into a fitness guru, run a marathon and lose fifty pounds overnight.

In my initial consultation I have a sheet filled with questions and statements for the client to fill out. Some of the things that I ask them to list are some of their short term and long term goals. An example of a realistic short term goal would be for a sedentary person to say that they would like to start walking 2-3 times a week for 30 minutes. That is a realistic doable goal to set and one that can most likely be met. An example of an unrealistic short term goal for a sedentary person would be to run a full marathon one month from now. That goal in itself will set you up for failure. It would be physically impossible to achieve and would eventually take a mental toll on you. Believe me you would not be able to go from sitting around doing nothing to running 26 miles in one month.

Ideally you want to set some realistic short term goals as well as long term ones. Write them down and keep them in your journal or notebook as a constant reminder of where you would like to get to. If you weigh 300 pounds and as a long term goal you would like to lose 100 pounds write it down and focus on it. If you work hard to do what it takes to lose those 100 pounds you will be able to look back and on it and see where you have met that specific goal. Then it will be time to set new ones because as you will learn goals are forever changing. Just make sure that when you are choosing goals that they are obtainable ones. If the goals that you have set for yourself seem unreachable you will be destined for failure and disappointed. Disappointment the majority of the time causes you to lose faith in the process and quit. So set your realistic long and short term goals write them down and get to them.

BABY STEPS

A baby does not come out of the womb walking and talking. These things are taught and learned by them as time passes. Just as in the new healthy lifestyle that you have chosen there are many things that you must learn. I will be the first one to admit that underneath the surface there is a lot of information and most of it in the beginning for you will be very confusing to say the least. It will take awhile before it will all make sense to you. Its relevance will not be revealed to you at first. That is why I you should take baby steps at the start.

We cannot expect that after many years as a couch potato that we can magically to turn into a fitness guru loving fitness right out of the gate. We don't all of a sudden love getting up way before it's time to go in for work to get our necessary workout time in. That miracle might not ever happen. Just because we take the steps to change our lives does not mean we automatically love it NOW. I will tell you right now that I absolutely hate doing cardiovascular training, but I love the way that it makes me feel. I can breathe better, dance longer, and surprisingly I have more energy. I have found something in it that pushes me to keep doing it day after day.

Start out slowly and build on things that you like or at least find interesting or intriguing. Change things in your life gradually taking it one day at a time. You should add and subtract things as your will power gets stronger. We pretty much know the things that are not healthy for us but with years of abusing our bodies with it, it is most times almost impossible to break those bad habits just like that. Removing all of the bad habits completely from our lives will take time, patience and lots of effort.

It is a lifestyle change in which we all start off as if we are newborn babies, learning a little something new adding to its everyday. We won't always be perfect, but if we look at each day is a new start it will help us hold it together. If you have fallen off the wagon, don't give up. Recognize your triggers and try to work on them for tomorrow. One step at a time, not big giant leaps.

Most people want to fly out of the gate because they feel they are behind in the race but doing this will cause you to burn out quickly and give up. You do not want to feel like becoming healthy is a chore so as I like to put it you must crawl before you walk. It is not a putdown or a slap back to you it is just getting you to add gradually, new and foreign things into your life. If you do it this way it becomes a part of your life and not something that you feel is a difficult task. Then it will become a complete lifestyle change.

Here are 10 simple things that you can gradually add into your life:
- *Take the steps instead of the elevator. This adds extra walking into your life without thought.*
- *Park further away from the store to get those extra steps into your day.*
- *Take a walk after lunch or after dinner. This will*

help burn calories as well as get your important steps in for the day.

- *Buy a pedometer. A pedometer is a small device that keeps count of your steps. You want to try to get 10,000 steps in per day. All the walking listed above will help you in achieving that goal.*

- *Take in smaller meal portions. America's food portion sizes have gotten too large. The right portions can make or break your progress. You want your potions to be no larger than the palm of your hand and no taller than a deck of playing cards.*

- *Drink plenty of water. Water helps to flush out toxins from the body and helps to speed up metabolism. It also helps give you the feeling of fullness to help combat over eating and keep you hydrated. Plus it has zero calories.*

- *Divide your meals into 5-6 small ones throughout the day. This helps stabilize your metabolism to help burn stored fat.*

- *Try to eat every 2-3 hours. This also helps to speed up metabolism. Try not to go longer than 4 hours before eating your next meal. This will keep blood sugar levels stable.*

- *In every meal you need a source of healthy protein, Healthy carbohydrate, and a source of healthy fat. Ex: Protein: lean meats, Carbohydrate: brown rice, Fats: almonds. Just remember potion control!*

- *Try to get in 30 minutes of exercise 3- 5 days a week. Exercise helps to burn stored fat and is also beneficial for your heart.*

GET EDUCATED, KNOWLEDGE IS POWER

Ok let's face it when wanting to do anything you must educate yourself about the topic that you have shown interest in. There is no possible way that you are able to know magically about something if you have not somewhat studied up on it. Now I am not saying to take college 101 courses in order for you to get started on your health and fitness journey but what I am saying to you is to at least know the basic necessary steps that enable you to get where you want to go.

There is nothing fancy involved and there are no magic tricks asked of you. My advice is for you to get the very basic knowledge that is out there for you. You do not have to buy every fitness book that has ever been written, nor do you have to surround yourself with the most difficult to understand information to succeed. Simplify the information as you start out. Nutrition and exercise does not have to be complex in order for it to work. Getting healthy has been the same since the beginning of time. The basic formula has not changed.

Gaining helpful knowledge is closer and less costly than you think. There is very helpful information offered to you in various places. If the internet is available to you it will be able to help you find such things as basic food groups, Basic exercises for beginners, and small lifestyle changes that you can incorporate into your life. Be very careful when searching for information on the internet because a lot of information is out there to sell a product or a service. You want to go to the medical pages that are set up on the internet to help you when you are seeking valid information. The library and your doctor's office is also a great place to seek out basic valuable information on beginning a healthy lifestyle. These places will likely have the information that is kept simple and broken down for you.

Avoid Information Overload

Sometimes too much of a good thing is a bad thing. In the beginning stages it is easy to gather too much information. We figure the more information that is gathered the better. This cannot be farther from the truth. How many times have we tried to listen to too many people and ended even more confused than ever? The problem is that a lot of the information that is written is written for different fitness levels. The things that I am able to understand and comprehend, a beginner might not have a clue of what is being talked about.

Yes we need guidance as we begin our journeys but we sabotage ourselves when we try to incorporate too many things all at once. It causes confusion and that will then lead to frustrations that will eventually cause you to quit. For the most part, everyone is saying the same thing in a different way. It is likely the same information, but just worded or presented in a different manner. So as a beginner it will not seem as such so the information will run all together and might not make any sense to you. A common mistake made by many is the infamous information overload.

My advice to you would be to like I stated in the previous chapter is to keep the information simplified. Also I would like to stress to you to follow one thing at a time. If you have found Jane Doe's information to be conducive and productive to your lifestyle then you need to follow her advice and stick to that only. It becomes too much when you try to incorporate too many people's advice into your world. You must give Jane Doe's program a chance to work for you. If you have find that it has not worked for you after you have worked hard and been consistent then by all means seek out more suitable information for you. But to keep down confusion and frustration is always to use one program at a time.

PUT OTHERS ON NOTICE

This step on the surface might not seem like a very important step but trust me it is a necessary one. Let's face it we have not lived our lives as healthy as we needed to for the most part. So when we make the decision to begin to change it for the better we must tell others around us. We have to remember that people around us have not made that same change that we have .They are used to us eating whatever we feel like eating, drinking like a fish, and hanging out at all times of the night. All these things definitely will not fit into your new healthy lifestyle. You will not progress if you keep these things in your life so therefore you must tell everyone that has influence in your life of the decision that you have made.

To start put your family, your friends, your co-worker, your church members and whomever else you feel should know about this change on notice. You want to alert them that you are starting your fitness journey because it does several helpful things for you. It lets them know that at this time you will no longer make the disastrous eating choices that you have made in the past. By letting them know what your plans are they are less likely to offer you that whole Red Velvet Cake that they made special for you. For the most part they will try to help you even if they have not made the choice to help themselves.

My experience has been that sense everyone in my circle knows my lifestyle they to make sure that I am comfortable when I am around them. If I am invited to a party of a close friend the host knows to have some healthy eating choices there for me. The same goes for the rare occasion that I go to a restaurant to eat with someone in my circle there is much thought and consideration when making a restaurant selection. All this is possible because I told them of my new lifestyle and how I strive to stick to it at all cost. If the people truly love you they will honor your wishes and will not try to knock you off track.

it then it becomes an almost tangible object to you. Many people have started their journeys far worse than yours and have gained success. We all started from somewhere but it all starts with mentally seeing what we desire to become.

HAVE A PLAN

Having a plan is critical to making a change in your life. Planning is the foundation on which everything is built upon. In everything that we do in order for there to be success we must have a plan. If we were building a building or teaching a class, there are plans of action that are thought out and written out. How can we expect or accept anything less when it comes to our most valuable asset, our bodies.

Setting a plan of action after you have decided to make healthier lifestyle changes will help you so far in succeeding on your journey. Sitting down and consciously writing down the steps that you plan to take will serve as a road map for your new life. It starts after you have done a previous step of writing your goals down. You have that information recorded, but how do you plan to get there? Having a plan will consist of you knowing and recording your workout times, the times that you plan to eat, as well as scheduling your rest time.

Planning all of these things is very essential to your success. Take some time out to sit down and plan out times and days that you can 100% devote yourself to these things. You know through your short term goal list that you would like to work out 3-5 times a week, so how do you plan to get there? Make it a habit to plan out the days and times that work best for you. Also try your best to keep that scheduled date and time. It is very important to do meal planning as well. Never wait until the last minute to figure out what and when you are going to eat. Life is not always on a time schedule I know, but if you plan ahead it will seem as if it is.

We might not think of rest as being part of getting healthy, but believe me it is. Not getting enough sleep will stagger our health efforts every time. Not getting enough rest will interfere with our energy levels in our workouts as well as throw our eating schedule way off track. With getting enough rest it requires us to go back to childhood and schedule a bedtime. Try your best to honor that bedtime every day and be strict when it comes to sticking to it. Begin to wind down an hour before your nightly set bedtime. At this time allow very few distractions to get in the way of your rest. Turn the television off and let the room be completely dark. If the telephone is a distraction turn the ringers off or on vibrate. Your body needs rest for it to function properly. This works for me because like the previous chapter states, I have already put everyone on notice about my bedtime schedule so as a rule I always turn my phone off after I am in bed so my sleep will not be disturbed.

Having a plan is always a great thing to incorporate into your life. Without a plan you won't know which way to go. You will know what you want but will have no idea of how you are going to get there. Having a plan also in a way holds you accountable for your actions. Look at your written plan as very important homework that you must get done to pass to the next grade.

Finding Motivation —

Sometimes as human being in order to get our motors running we must find some sort of motivation. I am not quite sure why we are wired that way but I say use whatever you have to use to get you focused and up off of the couch. Being a Personal Trainer I have heard some strange as well as not so strange reasons why a person wants to start their fitness journey. I have heard many get motivated because they are going on vacation. There is of course the wedding dress motivation. I personally like the 10th or 20th class reunion motivation. I have also heard a lot of the turning 40 or 30 vows to get fit and healthy. My all time favorite is doing it for another person. This one is done after a break up and the person decides there is no better revenge than looking great. There is also the worst one of all, the dreaded doctor's orders motivation. Kind of like get in better health or you will not be around too much longer.

I say whatever your motivation is use it to get started! If you are fighting for your life, when that clock goes off at 5am in order for you to get up and do your mornings walk, keep that in the front of your mind and use it as your motivation to get up and get moving. If you are nursing a broken heart use those emotions to select better food choices exercising smaller portions. If visualizing how great you are going to look if and when you see your ex again, use that mental picture to push you. Use any excuse to keep you motivated. Motivations change frequently but if it keeps you going I say by all means use them until you are able to say that fitness and proper nutrition is a permanent part of your life. It will give you something to strive and reach for. Remember don't stop keep going even if you have to find something else that will motivate you to keep moving.

REMOVE DISTRACTIONS

The facts are that we live in a fast paced world in which time waits for no one. That is the main reason we must remove the distractions from our lives. Distractions come in many forms. It can come from family, friends or frie-enemies, our jobs, a love affair, our kids, television shows, ECT. The list is endless and filled with things that can and will deter us from reaching our goals. Life is difficult and we can find any excuse to fall off of the fitness and good nutrition wagon. The key is to make you the priority. Be selfish when it comes to you and your health. It is not easy at first, but you are worth every bit of the struggle.

You are going to find that as soon as you make the effort to become healthier you will be faced with many distractions that are designed to throw you off track. Many people are emotional eaters so if they are going through unnecessary stress in their lives it will cause you to make bad food choices and then we tend to eat more of it. Jobs can cause a lot of distractions. Yes by all means do your job and do it well but if doing all of the extra things that are not in your job description causes you to stumble just remember that if you are not healthy you won't be able to effectively do your job anyway. The same goes for at home stresses that cause diversions. You have already put everyone on notice of your lifestyle change so now it is time to ask for help. Your family needs you healthy. You are able to do more for them when you are.

Television is the main distraction that will ruin us if we let it. It is almost as if it hypnotizes us and puts us in a trance. I truly believe that it makes us very lazy. We will get so distracted by the television that we will change plans that we made before hand to go to the gym. We have to realize that the people that we are watching and are so mesmerized by are living their lives so we must go and live ours. Instead of living our lives we tend to want to live vicariously through the television personality. There are only a few hours in the day so after you have come home from a hard day's work don't get distracted by what's on the television. It becomes important to use your time wisely. We only get one life to live and hopefully it will be a full one.

The biggest distractions in my opinion are people and relationships. For an example you will have your old party buddies who refuse to let you change your life for the better try to get you to go back to your old lifestyle. They will try and convince you that your old life can fit with your new one. Trust me, it does not. In your old life you ate maybe one time a day, eating anything that was available, you got about 3 hours of sleep a night and you sat on the couch watching countless hours of television. In your new lifestyle in order to achieve success all of that must die. Yet there are some that will try to entice you to return back to your old sluggish, lack luster, constipated, lifestyle. These are distractions that will get you off of your journey. You will begin to wonder why you stopped making progress. It is kind of like the scripture in the bible about not being able to serve two masters. You can't party all night and get up the next day to live a healthier lifestyle. Not to say that you can't ever party but everything in moderation and using discretion.

Lastly is relationship distraction. Being in a bad relationship whether it is a platonic friendship or a love affair can stop you dead in your tracks. It will cause you to overstress, forget your plans, overeat, neglect your workouts, not get enough or get too much rest, and lose your focus. If the relationship is draining and causing you to lose sight of what you are trying to accomplish then it is nothing more than a distraction. When this is happening it is time for you to move on to more positive beginnings. You must not allow anything to come between you and your health.

BE CONSISTENT WITH YOUR NEW LIFESTYLE

Consistency is the key to your success. You must make fitness and nutrition a part of your life and stay consistent in order to see results. You are not likely to see results with sporadic good eating habits and workouts. Fitting them both into your life on a regular basis will give you the results that you seek. As a trainer I have had many clients that would like to have the results they seek yesterday but they will miss appointments and eat fast food everyday for at least two of their meals. That is not the type of consistency needed to change your life. Real results are brought by real consistent change.

Sticking to your scheduled gym time, your meal planning and keeping a consistent sleep schedule will propel you to what you always knew you could be. Set up a time and stick to it as closely as possible. Look at this time as if it were a job. Don't call in unless it is absolutely necessary. Your results most definitely will not happen overnight. But in time and being able to stick to a good plan on a consistent basis it will happen. You will begin to notice gradual small changes that will give you the mental push you need in order to keep going. Stick to your plans and follow your schedule by any means necessary.

PREPARATION

When it comes to getting healthy there is only one word that will help you reach your goals time after time and that word is preparation. Your new lifestyle requires a lot of planning. You must plan a time to work out, plan your meals, and also as already stated plan to get enough sleep.

Since I don't work on Sundays, I plan and cook my meals for that upcoming week. Freezer bags and a good set of Tupperware will become your best friend. If you are going to be out for the day take your food and snacks with you to avoid eating out at unhealthy fast food places. Invest in a medium sized to large cooler to store your items in. Keep in mind that there are no vending machines with carrot sticks and hummus and there are hardly any places that you can just pull into that won't get you off of your nutrition plan, so you must be prepared at all times. If you plan to be out for the entire day pack enough nutritious meals and snacks to last you throughout the day. This helps you to stick to the plan more effectively. It is also cheaper on your wallet in the long run.

Preparation is not only in preparing food but with everything. You must plan the time that you are going to work out and stick to it! If we deviate from our planned time we know it likely will not happen for that day. We are creatures of habits and any diversion will cause our minds to stray. So stay prepared so there are no surprises to knock you off of your horse.

RANDOM HELPFUL TIPS

Buy a timeless outfit that you just love, but don't buy it in your current size; buy it in the size that you desire to be. (But, remember to be realistic) Hang the dress in a place where you are able to see it every day. This will serve as a constant reminder to you of your goals you have set for yourself. Mentally it will help you stay on track until it all becomes second nature to for you.

You should purchase a trip for 6 months to a year out (depending on where you are in your fitness and nutrition life) to a wonderful place that you have always wanted to go, hang the ticket where you can see it often. Visualize the new you on that beach, or wherever your destination may be. If you have a class reunion approaching it would be great to shock everyone at that reunion so plan ahead. These thoughts can motivate and propel you through.

Find a picture of someone that you strive to be like physically. It can even be an old picture of how you used to look. Take that picture and hang it somewhere that you go to often. It can be hung in the bathroom, the car mirror visor, or on the refrigerator. Just make sure it is hung somewhere that you look at several times a day. Use the photo as a reminder to stay focused when you look at it.

Have your alarm clock wake you up with a motivational tune. Select something that when you hear it will remind you that you have made a promise to yourself to really focus and commit this time. Pick something that will inspire you to get up and get moving. Alarm clocks on cell phones are great for this. You can download almost any song to your cell phone and program it to go off at the time you chose.

As soon as you return from the market prepare your foods. You can wash and clean all of your fruits and vegetables. You can also boil your entire carton of eggs that they are accessible to you when you need them the most.

FOOD IS NOT THE ENEMY

The sooner we realize that food is not the enemy the better. We must realize that our relationship with food is in most cases a major problem. The different ways that we view food will determine if our journey will become a success or failure. I was raised to always clean my plate because I was told by my mother that we didn't have any food to waste. Sorry Mom, but that became embedded into my head even as an adult, to always finish everything that was on my plate even if I was stuffed. I did not want to be wasteful so I ate and ate until it was all gone, always. It wasn't until later on in life that I realized that the simple statement that was made to me so many years ago was the reason for me wanting to always overeat. I finally figured that one out so now I put only small portions on my plate (Remember palm size of hand and as tall as a deck of card) So look mom I am not being wasteful.

Sometimes we tend to eat out of emotions. We eat if we are stressed, sad, happy, bored, and so on. Knowing that food is not the problem but it is more so not controlling our portions and the kinds of food that we are eating is what plagues us. I know if we are sad the last thing we want to eat is a celery stick with natural peanut butter on it. Our bodies will crave the bad fat. But keep in mind that this is only a temporary high that will more than likely lead to you feeling even worse plus it might leave you with a side of guilt. We tend to want to associate food with everything and with every occasion. When you are feelings stressed and have already had your meal go for a walk instead of raiding the refrigerator. You should call and speak with a friend. Make sure that it is a positive friend that you can just let it all hang out with. Or maybe you can go window shopping to help get your emotions back in order.

We must analyze our relationship with food. Find out if it is a good or bad relationship. Check to see if we are an emotional eater and find out our triggers. Look for other ways to calm ourselves and regain control. Also remember it is okay not to finish all of your food. If you are full your body will let you know it so there is no need to continue to eat. We want to start "eating to live" not "living to eat"

NEVER STARVE YOURSELF TO LOSE WEIGHT

There is a misconception that to lose weight you must starve yourself. This is one of the biggest falsehoods ever told. Our bodies need food to survive. Starvation diets cause a host of other health issues in the long run. I always use the analogy that our bodies are our vehicles and we cannot run our cars without gas in them. Food for our bodies is our gas. If you deprive yourself of food we get sluggish, run down and eventually shutdown. Not taking in enough food will cause your body to burn precious lean muscle for fuel. Our lean muscle is used to burn stored fat. With less and less of lean muscle, it makes it almost impossible to lose weight later. So you might lose weight at first and quick I might add, because you have lost more than just fat. You have lost muscle as well and with less muscle it makes it difficult to combat stored and future fat.

Ideally we would like our bodies to become fat burning machines and trust me if you work hard it will. Like a vehicle the better quality of things that you use to keep it going the better, the same is true with our bodies. So of course changing the type of food that we choose to put into our bodies will make it run much better, but until we are able to get to that point all that is needed is to cut back. If we remember our portion sizes, redefine of relationship with food, and listen to our bodies we will have success without starvation.

Give your taste buds time to adjust

Ok it is always so easy to say what you do not like. Sometimes we say that we don't like it before we have tried it. That is to me a cop out. I know that there are something's that are great for you that will be unpleasant to your taste buds. I am not saying to eat those things .You will not just magically enjoy all things healthy. But I am saying to you to have an open mind and be willing to try different things. I am not asking you to clear out all of your favorite things and replace it with all healthy items because you probably won't like all of them. I don't like all of them, but just try them and begin to replace healthy items for your unhealthy ones one by one.

It will take time for our taste buds to readjust. After which you still will not love everything but the key is to find the ones that you do like, use them and begin to add to them. Instead of seasoning foods with the usual added fats, try seasoning foods with other foods. If you normally cook things in butter use low sodium chicken broth and other vegetables such as onions and bell peppers. It is a definite change and your taste buds might recognize it, but at least you are trying new things to maybe experience something you like. A lot of times you will find that the changes will be subtle and can almost go unnoticed. These changes are needed and much healthier for you.

As we age we need a certain amount of vitamins and minerals for our bodies to function properly and it is most desirable to get them from our food sources. Our meal plans should not look like a toddler's or a college student. Not that theirs should either, but aging should be a critical pivotal moment in our lives that begin to change our eating habits if haven't already. If we are patient with our taste buds giving them time to change we will reap the rewards physically.

Change your eating habits before starting your workouts

Often times when deciding to live a healthy Lifestyle the first thing that we do is start to work out. We join a gym, get a workout partner or start walking or running. In my professional opinion I think that doing so is the one of the worst things that you could do. If you are not under the guidance of a nutritionist or Dietian understanding food and its benefits will be the first thing that you will need to do. Working out comes natural for our bodies so it is so easy to jump into that and adjust. The hard part is reversing 20, 30 or 40 plus year's worth of bad eating habits.

The truth of the matter is that you can lose weight without exercise but I do not advise that. I feel that having good nutrition and exercise work together is more beneficial to your overall health. I recommend getting your eating habits started first because it gives your body a chance to detoxify and adjust. It won't seem so overwhelming if you do this first. If you would like to walk or jog while doing this by all means do so.

If you plan to go all in and do the entire eating healthier lifestyle change or even if you plan to just try to control your portions then you will need give your body time to adjust to the change. After the grocery store trip, which I will talk about later, I like to tell my clients to take about a week to just focus on incorporating great nutrition into their lives. It is a lot to deal with especially if you are totally clueless about what it involves to make the necessary changes. In which most cases we all are clueless about it at some point. Telling them to do this takes a lot of the unnecessary stress away while they transition.

KEEP A FOOD JOURNAL

Keeping a Food Journal will be very beneficial to you. Keeping a record of everything that goes into your mouth does several things for you. One of those things is that it allows you to know exactly how much you are eating. If you are overeating as well as under eating, keeping an accurate account of this will show exactly that. Sometimes unless written out we will not be able to believe how many calories that we are consuming. So if it is in black and white we are then able to sit down and figure out we can make some cuts in calories or in some cases add a few.

A food journal will also keep you honest with yourself. As crazy as it sounds when we start on our journeys we will lie to ourselves about what and how much we really eat. Lying to ourselves will only hurt us in the long run. Our Food Journals should be private and unless under a physician, nutrition list, or dietician's orders should be for our eyes only. So to lie in the pages of your food journal would be senseless and hurtful to you.

A food Journal can also serve as a reference to you. I like to put small stars by delicious meals that I enjoyed. I do this in order to recreate that dish at a later date. If the meal was not so enjoyable I draw a small arrow pointing downward by expressing that I might need to tweak the recipe a little bit.

There are journals made especially for this but you can also make your own out of a plain tablet. When making your own please date it, record the time and what meal it was. At the end of the day you can go to the computer and find several sites that offer free calorie counters in order to record and calculate your calories for the day. If don't have internet access there are several books and electronics available that count daily calories.

HAVE A MEAL PLAN

In an earlier lesson the importance of being prepared was stressed. This lesson speaks about having a meal plan which goes right along with being prepared. Having a meal plan is just half of the equation that I spoke about. The other half of the equation is manifesting that meal plan. Each week in your spare time, you should sit down and write out your meals for at least 5 days. If you are like a lot of people you have the weekend off. Use one of those days to prepare your meals planned for that week. I use Sunday as my day to do this. Instead of cooking just enough chicken breast and veggies for that day I cook the entire package or enough to cover all of the days that I put chicken breast on my menu. Some of your best friends will be storage containers, baggies and aluminum foil.

I know that a lot of people will cringe at this step because they despise leftovers. That is when I ask them to ask themselves what's important to you. It is about changing your life and not about doing the same old thing because that has not worked for you. Not having a meal ready and cooked for you after you come home from a long day at work is not a good thing. Picture this, you are hungry (which means you have waited too long to eat anyway) tired and now you have to cook yourself a meal.

While you are cooking I guarantee that you would have eaten up half of the food in the kitchen before your meal is finished. Doing this leads to extra unrecorded calories. When we have calories that we have not accounted for results in no weight being lost or worse a weight gain so on the surface it makes it look as if the process does not work.

The process does work you just failed to plan. If you fail to plan then you might as well plan on failing. Having a meal plan is crucial to your success. With every great success there must be a plan. Have your meal plan, cook them up, and store them to turn your body into the fat burner that it was meant to be.

Shop in the "U Shape" in the Grocery Store

Have you ever noticed that no matter what grocery store you are in, the healthiest of the foods are located along the U Shape of it? Did you notice that the unhealthiest food is in the middle? The U Shape is the side area in the front that travels along the back side and goes up and around again the back side of the grocery store. You have the beginning side with fruits and vegetables. You are always welcome there. The back of the U is where you should look for your lean meats such as chicken breast, lean fish, and lean beef. On your way back up the other side of the U is where you should look for your low fat dairy products such as your low fat milk, low fat cheeses, low fat yogurts and your eggs. Most of the time on the opposite side you will find your frozen vegetables (without sauces of course) If you think of that as a U and do the majority of your shopping in that "U" then you will gain much success.

Choose foods that are as close to their natural state as possible

When you are choosing foods to eat you want to stick to the ones that are as close to the natural state as possible. Your body recognizes these foods so it makes the processes from digestion to elimination much easy. Foods that are in their natural state also have many needed vitamins and minerals in them. With foods that are processed a lot of the important nutrients are stripped away. We can supplement to help our food out buy getting on a regimen of manufactured vitamins but whenever possible try to get the majority of your vitamins and mineral from food sources.

Examples of some foods left in their natural state are vegetables, fruit, natural nuts, and unprocessed meats. When selecting items try to choose foods described as *plain, raw or in its own juices.* So if you were choosing a frozen bag of peas it would be best to get the bag that ingredients state *Peas.* Try not to get it in butter or sauces. That adds unnecessary fat as well as calories. Sometimes you might come out better by just eating something unhealthy compared to eating an *advertised* healthy product drenched in sauces. Another not so great choice is canned goods. I know that canned goods are easier on the pocketbook but the sodium per serving is way too high on most of them. Too much sodium can lead to high blood pressure which can cause heart attack or stroke.

FAMILIARIZE YOURSELF WITH FOOD LABELS AND FOOD INGREDIENTS

As a consumer the best thing that you can do is to familiarize yourself with food labels and their ingredients. On the back or side of every item there is a label that will tell you all of that particular foods nutrition fact. It tells you the calories, total fat grams per serving size, the sodium content, protein percentage, carbohydrate percentage, and the vitamins and minerals added. Sometimes there are a lot of other ingredient percentages as well. Each food item will tell you how many servings you are able to get from that one product. At times it is 2 or 3 so if you eat the entire box you must multiply the calories by 2 or 3 to get the accurate amount of calories that were consumed. Read those labels to determine your numbers in order to keep an accurate account.

It is also very conducive to your new lifestyle to go one step further by reading the ingredients that are listed on the label. Keep in mind that companies are in business and their main job is to market their product and sell it to the consumer whether it is good, bad, or indifferent. Just because the company says that it is good for you does not mean that it is. Do you think that they would tell you that it is terrible for your health? No. They simply could not afford to do so because it would bankrupt them. So that is why it is important to gain your own knowledge and become a label and ingredient reader.

The fewer ingredients an item has, the better. That means it is more in its natural state and has been processed less. When food is processed a lot of the natural things have been taken out and replaced with manmade chemicals. They add these things to give their products a longer shelf life. When you read the ingredients, it should have names that you recognize and can understand without having to get a dictionary. Also the higher up in the ingredient list an item is, the more the product has of it. So if a can of soda pop's list reads: *Water, sugar, high fructose corn syrup, corn syrup* you can just stop right there and put that item back. That list just told me that it is just sugar water. So no matter how healthy, sugar or fat free they say it is always turn it over and read the label and the ingredient content. You will often find that the label will tell a different tale.

How Your Plate Should Look

Believe it or not there is a certain way your plate should look. Besides the portion control rule of thumb, your plate should be very colorful. Along with your lean protein and good carbohydrate you should fill your plate with lots colorful fruit and veggies. Vegetable and fruit have a lot of fiber in them which keeps us fuller longer and keeps things moving along in our digestion system. A small list of good colorful things that should be on your plate is:

Spinach ,collard greens,mustard greens,turnip greens, broccoli, Brussels sprouts, cabbage ,kale, peas, avocado, carrots, mangos, apricots, cantaloupes, pumpkin, squash ,sweet potatoes, cranberries, blueberries, blackberries, strawberries, red apples, grapes, orange juice, oranges, tangerines, peaches, papayas, nectarines, garlic, onions, celery and pears.

There are many others that you should work onto your plate. Try some out to find your flavor.

TRY TO DRINK LESS ALCOHOL

As I have already been told by my entire client list trying to drink less is easier said than done. This one topic is almost non negotiable when it comes to weight lose for a few reasons. It has no good nutritional value and is only in the food group by default. It is not really a food but in some studies it is listed as one. Alcohol is just a poison toxin to our bodies. It is comprised of mostly sugar and immediately turns to such as soon as it enters our bodies. For all of us there lies the bad news because it goes straight to our bellies. That is the last place we want it to go as a male or a female.

Drinking alcohol in my experience sometimes will cause you to make terrible food choices if we become inebriated. We stop thinking about what going into our bodies the moment that happens. We need to be able to make clear and level head choices. Also alcohol is full calories and fat we don't add it into our daily calorie counting. We ignore it as if it were calorie free. Let's face it a lot of us when it comes to having a drink do not know our limit. That is when the calories just keep adding up. Alcohol can worst of all throw our workout game off for sometimes weeks.

It has been said that having a daily glass of wine can help ward off certain cancers but some of us are all or none type people, which means we are not drinking red wine with the hopes of keeping us cancer free. And be honest most of us are not drinking wine anyway. So when it comes to this subject you might have to again choose what is important to you. I am not saying to you never to have a drink but I am saying to you like I have said to many of my clients you can have that drink every day.

PLAY WITH RECIPES

Hopefully when you get into your kitchen you will begin to play with different taste. You can find healthier options for grandma's chicken casserole recipe. You can even invent your own recipes once you establish what type of taste you like. In the beginning it might seem as if you are eating the same ole boring things. That is because this is a whole new experience for you and you don't know quite yet which direction to take your new healthy food journey in. I say get in there and experiment with different natural flavors in your spare time. If it doesn't come out right the first time if you have the time, money, interest and energy try it again at a later date.

I have made some of the best tasting recipes just by taking something that I used to make unhealthily and replacing those ingredients with healthy ones. I keep a note pad in the kitchen to record the ingredients and directions just in case I like it. I got tired of the same ole menu too but I did not want to give up on my healthy lifestyle so I decided to spice up my food with other foods. I have a few tasty recipes in the book that hopefully you will cook and enjoy for yourself. Maybe you will be able to change up my recipes adding or subtracting things to your liking.

RULES FOR EATING OUT

Yes there are rules to follow when you are eating out in a restaurant. I do realize that not everyone can cook or even have the desire to cook, but in order for this to work for you must adhere to a few rules when you do dine out. I would prefer that you bought all of your food from the grocery store and prepare all of your meals yourself but in the real world I realize that can't and won't always happen. So here are a couple of helpful tips for you when you dine out.

>*Pick a place where they have healthier choices.*

>*When ordering ask for your food to be cooked in little or no oil or butter. You can ask if steaming is an option. Don't be afraid to do this. With obesity becoming out of control the world is slowly coming around so they will understand.*

>*Keep in mind that most restaurants have portions so ask if you can half already boxed away in a to go box and brought out to you when you are ready to leave.*

> *Ask for no sauce and dressing on the side if you insist on having it.*

>*Order water to drink. This will help fill you up, keep the fiber moving and it is zero calories or fat.*

>*If allowed order the kids meal. It is usually the correct portion size for an adult.*

> *Try not to go to a buffet. There is just too much temptation there.*

> *If you can help it try not to go to a restaurant when you are in an emotionally funk. All of your good eating habits will probably go out of the window on that day.*

> *Eat slowly. This gives your food time to digest giving your brain enough time to get the signal that you are full.*

>*Bring your food journal along with you. If have purchased a calorie counter book or electric calorie counter bring it along as well. Most menus don't list the caloric measurement.*

>*Keep the colorful, well portioned plate in mind. A lot of restaurants are adding healthier choices to their menus.*

> *If you are full then stop eating! Ask for a to- go box, Give it away or leave there right on the table.*

Rules for dinner parties, Bar-b-Qs, Family gatherings

The fact is that we don't all change at the same time. Just because you have decided on a healthier lifestyle does not mean that everyone else is going to do the same thing. At this year's gatherings expect to see the same kinds of foods being served that were served in the past. You have to prepare yourselves for these types of situations. The key is to make it out without being all the way turned back into your old selves.

We all can agree that fatten foods are delicious as well as addictive. Sometimes we are not close to being hungry but we still will grab something that looks delicious to snack on. To help combat this try eating one of your meals before you go. When you are tempted you are able to tell yourself unequivocally that you are not hungry and that you just see it and want it. Find something else to do that doesn't revolve around food. You can also bring nuts as a snack with you. If you find yourself getting hungry before it is time snack on a few raw almonds or walnuts. I find that if I don't stand too close to the food, I am not as tempted. Lastly, if you are comfortable enough to do this, bring your own meals. There are times that there won't be anything for you to eat so be prepared and bring your own meals. Everyone there will know your lifestyle so they won't be offended by it. You can even make a healthy dish to serve. Sometimes we can rub off on them instead of it being the other way around.

TREAT YOURSELF

TO ONE CHEAT MEAL

PER WEEK

Saying this to some of us is like saying to a drug addict that it is ok to get high one time per week. Admittedly some of us cannot handle going back to the fattening foods on a weekly basis. But this helps us out mentally as well as physically. When we feel deprived we most likely will not stick to our new lifestyle. So let's say we plan to have our one cheat on Saturday when we are scheduled to go out to lunch with the family that will mentally motivate us to stick to the plan the entire week up until Saturday. We know we will be able to get that slice of devil food's cake that we so craved so we will nine times out of ten wait for that day to come to get that one meal that we have thought about.

For us physically, getting that one cheat meal will help balance out our calories. Sometimes while trying to lose weight we go under the amount of calories needed for our bodies. When we fail to keep an accurate food journal this can often time happen. Eating that one cheat meal may help boost the calories up to where they should be. Generally cheat meals are scheduled for earlier in the day in order to burn off most of the calories while you are awake.

Did you notice that I keep reintegrating "Cheat Meal"? I did that for a purpose. A client and a very dear friend of mine one entire month later came to me swearing that I told her that she could have a cheat day. So for an entire month she had just indulged herself in whatever she wanted to eat or drink for a whole day. An entire day can put you back at square one. Because of that situation I want to be clear about the rules of a cheat meal and they are as followed:

1. *A cheat meal is whatever meal that you chose being able to eat whatever you'd like. One meal, one time a week!*
2. *A cheat meal is to be consumed in that time frame in that one sitting. Whatever you do not finish is given away or goes in the trash.*
3. *As an example if I chose my cheat meal for lunch then for breakfast, dinner and one or two snacks are my normal healthy eating.*

Helpful Kitchen Tools that make your Healthy life easier

There are many helpful kitchen items that are on the market that will make your healthy journey easier. It is not necessary to run out and purchase all of these tools but a few of them are very essential in my opinion. Here is my list of favorite items that helped and still help me out in the kitchen listed in no particular order.

1. *A juicer: This is great when preparing your own fresh fruit and veggie juices. Instead of paying high cost for the store bought manufactured juices you can make your own at home fresh.*

2. *Steamer: This is a lifesaver for me. I am able to steam rice, veggies, and meats in a jiffy. Make sure you get one with a timer on it.*

3. *A powerful blender: I have found a marvelous blender that I never put away. I use it to make protein shakes, smoothies (for my sweet tooth), soups, chicken salad, and sorbet all from natural ingredients. Make sure you invest in a really good one.*

4. *Crock pot (slow cooker): I love crock pots because you can cook an entire meal without any attention.*

5. *Panini Maker: You can load your sandwiches up with vegetables with this machine. It presses them into a tight delicious sandwich.*

6. *Oven bags: These work great for busy people. You can add all of your ingredients into the bag close it and pop it into the oven with little or no attention*

7. *Lunchbox: This is very important for you to have when you are out and about. It will help to keep your meals hot or cold. You should plan ahead*

by packing your meals and take your lunch box
wherever you go.

8. *Zip lock bags: Use these to freeze foods to keep fresh
longer. They can also take the place of Tupperware
to take up less space.*

DON'T BEAT YOURSELF UP

In this journey there might be many times that you
unintentionally fall off of the wagon of health and fitness.
This will likely happen to you, but do not beat yourself
up. It happens to all of us. Life gets in the way sometimes
and it makes it very difficult to stay the course. If we beat
ourselves up over our misstep that gives way to quitting
altogether. The lesson here is to know that everyone falls
off of the Health Wagon at one point or another. Realize
now that everyone puts something in their mouths that
they shouldn't at some point or another, or misses an
occasional work out session. When this occurs don't
Waller in your missteps. When you mess up realize it and
recognize what caused that slip up. Think of what you
can do to not let it happen again too soon. Just because
you messed up for lunch does not mean your entire day
is destroyed. Pick yourself up and move forward in the
right direction. Tomorrow is a new day. Better yet the
next minute is a new start!

Revaluate
YOURSELF PERIODICALLY

In order to know if you are going in the right direction it is important to reevaluate yourself. When you do this you will be reevaluating your physical gains or lack of as well as how far you've come mentally. After I have completed an entire monthly evaluation which consist of me re-testing their weight, body fat percentage, blood pressure, measurements, and fit test I recommend to my clients to go home and write a list of things that they have changed for the better and things that they can change to further improve their journey. This is their personal journey information written for their records only. This can be written in your fitness book or your food journal. This will keep you focused on your future goals whether you saw improvements or if you did not. If you did not see any improvement then that is a perfect chance for you to write down things you can do in order to see some progression by your next monthly evaluation.

Be honest with yourselves

An important ingredient to your success is for you to be honest with yourself. Lying to yourself is one way to stop your progression. If we do not admit to our faults we will never make strides to try and change them. As impossible and silly as it sounds people do this all of the time. We lie about how much change we really have made and it holds us back from achieving what we want. We must sincerely admit to what we are or are not doing in order to see true change. It is easy to boast to friends about the changes we have made but did we really? Staying honest and true to you brings about changes.

Plan of action in the gym

I was at the gym one day trying to get a quick workout in before my client was scheduled to arrive. I had decided that today would be my day to work my back, biceps and forearms. I had everything mapped all out. The type exercises, the sets, the reps, and right up to an estimation of rest in between sets. Normally I am much focused, but that day I could not help but to notice something eye-catching while I was getting my 35- 40 minutes of hard intense training in. I noticed another lady in the gym whom I had never seen before working out as well. The lady was walking around aimlessly almost as if she was lost. She went from this machine to that one with a look of confusion all about her. The exercises were done randomly and without the proper form. I could tell just by looking at her that she felt lost and out of place.

I said all of that to say, HAVE A PLAN. Before you arrive at the gym you should already know what you are going to do. If it is a cardio day, stick to that. If it is leg day, do legs. Always have your routine ready to go.

Everyone can not afford a Personal Trainer, but there are other ways to skin a cat. I stated before that you can buy books, magazines or DVDS. If you are a member of a gym, take classes and mimic one of the routines that were done in the class while working out on your own. There are other reasons not talked about that people give up on their training. One of the reasons is that they feel out of place. The feelings go far beyond feeling completely uncomfortable. Often times as human beings instead of sticking it out until those feelings of awkwardness subside, we quit, and stop working out altogether.

Many people might have equipment in their homes, but that equipment eventually turns into clothes racks. This reigns true for a lot of the hard core, die hard people who work out as well. They find it very difficult to find the focus to work out at home. That takes a special determined person to do this consistently.

My advice is that if you have the money hire a trainer for a few months until you get the hang of things. That will help you especially if you are new to working out in a gym or even working out at home. A trainer can help you with proper form and technique to help you avoid injury and reach some of you goals quicker. Surely doing this is cheaper in the long run than paying the medical bills that you might incur. When you invest in this it will give you a less likely chance of getting hurt and continuing.

If you are short on money, go to a book store and find you a good workout book that will take you from point A to B. A good book would be one that explains the entire exercise from start to finish, exactly what it does and, what specifically what muscles that the exercise works. DVDS are great because you can see exactly what the person is doing while giving you directions verbally. Remember to follow one thing at a time. Too much information is overkill.

The bottom line is with everything that we do there is a plan to it. We have plans in our jobs, our schools, the way we run our households, and the list can go on. Exercise planning should not be any different. After all, we are planning to protect the most important investment that we have. That is our one and only body.

Sit down and determine what the plan is for that day and write it down. You can go as far as planning it out for the week if that helps you say on track. This will save you a lot of time and also will help to make your workout experience a more enjoyable one.

KEEP A WORKOUT JOURNAL

Just as you need to keep a food journal it is important to keep a workout journal as well. These books can be purchased at book stores or online. It is easiest that you purchase one because it is already set up for you. Keeping a workout journal will keep track of the exercises that you have done on any particular day. It is there to record what weight you lifted or pushed and how many times you did on a particular exercise. Later on when you are stronger you will be able to look back at how far you have come. It also is a great way of planning out your workouts. Like in the previous story that I spoke about it is so imperative that you have a plan of action before hand. Having a plan keeps you on a schedule and not wondering around aimlessly. When you do that aimless wonder you will burn out quick because of feelings of never belonging. I stated before with everything important there should be a written plan of action and there is nothing more important than your one life. So get one write your exercises down and take it with you when you workout.

DO THINGS THAT YOU HATE THE LEAST

It has been the hot question of my career so far and that is what kind of cardiovascular exercise I should do in order to lose weight. My answer to that question has always been to do the exercise that you love or at least hate the least. I must admit that I hate cardiovascular training. I love to weight train but if I could accomplish all what I wanted to accomplish with cardiovascular training I would not do it. Cardiovascular Training is physical conditioning that exercises the heart, lungs and the associated blood vessels. Examples of cardiovascular training is walking, jogging, running, boxing, dancing, riding a bike, & using machines such as elliptical, stair masters, step mills, Jacob's ladders. You can also do things such as playing a sport or activity. I hate all of the above with the exception of dancing, but we must do cardio in order to keep our hearts healthy and remove that unwanted stored fat.

So I tell my clients to test a few of the exercises out. I want them to determine which exercise works best for them. I would love for them to determine which one that they hate and not to do that one. My philosophy is the same way I feel about foods, if you hate it you won't do it. I am not saying that it will be the highlight of your day but if you are able to find something that you like about it then you are most likely going to do it. But if you dread it you will feel anxious and then you are not inclined to do it. I use dancing as my cardio because I love it. I hip hop dance, salsa, and a new one that I found to burn a lot of calories for me is a dance called Krumping. My son says no one does it anymore but it sure helps me burn a lot of calories. I do other kinds of cardiovascular training but this is the only one that that I look forward to. Try out different machines or activities and see which ones that you can live with and go out and do it at your pace. We have to do it so it might as well be something that we like.

Music makes you lose control

Trust me when I tell you that the first thing that you need to invest in is a good music player. Whatever brand that you chose is fine just making sure that you put some money into this one particular item. Having a music player has been so important to me thus far on my journey. Whether I am at the gym or have chosen to workout at home I have needed a music player. Besides the fact that I love music and any kind of music, having it handy while I train has propelled me to go further in my workouts. There have been times that I have turned my car around to return home at 3 am in the morning to retrieve my music player. Mentally I think I am unable to train without it.

Music can help you push past your level of comfort when used as a motivator or a distraction. Pick uplifting motivational music to download to your listening device. Also if you can choose a device that you can make playlist. This will allow you to strategically play the songs that you would like to hear back to back. There are many songs recorded old and new that seem as if were made to listen to while you workout. Find the type of music that speaks to your spirit in all genres. This will make your workouts seem to go faster and effortlessly. Hearing some particular songs can even push you to push harder or even finish that last repetition. At the end of these lessons I will list some of the songs that have helped me to push past my limits.

JOIN A GYM

If at all possible join a gym. I know that saying this to you right now in this economy might seem impossible but it is an investment in your biggest and best asset, you. For some this might seem like a stretch and a little out of reach but you cannot afford to not do this. Most gyms nowadays have many specials and reduced prices to get you started. They are practically begging people to come in and join. I have run across gyms offering $10 a month for monthly fees. If you add up all of the money that you waste on things that have no value or purpose I am sure that you can handle $10 a month. Now divided that cost by 30 days and see how reasonable the cost is to you. You might be able to pay in full at prices that low. It would be worth it to do so.

Joining a gym has great value. If you join a gym you are more likely to work out on a regular basis than people who do not. It takes a strong person to workout at home, but if you have a gym membership it is as if you have an appointment to go to. It gets you out of the house meeting and greeting other like mind individuals. Also a lot of gyms will give free gym orientations showing you how equipment works and what body parts they train. Some also offer free nutrition advice and offer group classes. By joining a gym it says that you are not going at it alone because you can always ask for assistance. Nowadays a lot of the gyms are throwing in a lot of extras to lure you into joining their club. Look into prices and perks for gyms and fitness centers in your area. It will be your best help when starting out.

JOIN IN ON GROUP FITNESS CLASSES

As in the previous lesson I encouraged you to join a gym to propel you in your new lifestyle. If you are able to do so try to participate in some of the group fitness classes that are offered. Most of these classes are offered free to the members so all you need to do is show up. Some facilities extend the classes to non members as well. They are normally done on a schedule and run throughout the day and evening. These classes are an inexpensive way to better fitness. They can also be motivation for you if you are competitive or need that extra push because you can take them with a family member or a friend. There are many great classes offered from muscle building and sculpting classes to fat burning ones. There are a lot of fun dance classes to attend like hip hop, salsa, jazz and combination dance classes. Some gyms or fitness facilities offer stretching and yoga classes which are very important to your fitness. If you are unable to join a gym on a regular basis check out classes offered in your area. Some of these are on a pay as you go system but my advice is not to go this route if you can help it. Typically you opt not to go if you have not paid for it in advance than if you already have paid. Think about it and then you decide which works best for you.

Get a workout partner

A good piece of advice to you is to get a workout partner. Find someone that is just a little bit ahead of the game than you. Finding a more advanced partner will push you further than if you have one that is on the same level as you. A workout partner who has incorporated fitness into their life a little longer than you is more inclined to go and workout when it is time to do so. In some cases two people on the same fitness level will make excuses for not going to train on that day. Sometimes neither one of the beginners will have the will power to stand up and say yes we will push through go today. Their excuses will seem to make sense collectively.

There are many places to look for a workout partner. If you are a member of a gym you can post a want ad on the bulletin board. Sometimes if you ask around in your church there are people that will be delighted to mentor you in your journey. They can look not too far back and remember what it was like when they first started out. Sometimes being a mentor to you will motivate them. You can also put out an ad in the personals if you feel comfortable doing that. But please be careful when going this route. It has worked out great for some people though. A workout partner at any level can be great if that is what you desire.

HIRE A PERSONAL TRAINER

Ok obviously this lesson is on a *do this if you can basis*. I am stating this not because I myself am a Personal Trainer, but because there are a lot of reasons that you should hire a Personal Trainer. When you have been ordered by a doctor to lose weight because of health reasons, it becomes very important time to hire a Personal Trainer. Most Trainers can help you reach you goals in half of the time that you can by doing it by yourself. Trainer's have knowledge of what level to keep your heart rate in order to lose. We also keep you safe with performing a particular exercise. Sometimes you cannot, not afford to hire one because it is a life or death situation.

Another situation when it is important to hire a Personal Trainer would be when you have a massive amount of weight to lose. Even if you have to hire a Trainer on a temporary basis I would recommend that you do so. This will help you in gaining a little knowledge when first starting. If you can afford to keep them on then by all means do so. It will be beneficial to you. If you find yourself at a plateau (a standstill) with your fitness this is a great time to locate and interview possible trainers. They will be able to get you pass your stand still point with new innovative training. You should be able to tell the difference with their workouts and your own.

Many people are fearful of Trainers and their cost or they just feel that they are capable of doing it on their own. My answer to that is not in the beginning you most likely are not. No matter the costs realize that you are your best asset and if you're is too sick that might end it all. Sometimes it cost to repair what we have destroyed and if that means doing your research and interviewing a potential trainer to hire then do it. This will take a lot of burden off of you with everything dealing with your new lifestyle. They will be able to help you with your workout with them as well as outside of them and your nutrition. If you look at all of the great athletes they all have Trainers. That person has studied that particular thing to get you where you need to go.

As far as pricing do not be afraid of inquiring because just as I stated in the Join a gym lesson there is a lot of deep discounting being offered in this troubled economy. A lot of Trainers are offering package deals and group rates for 2-3 people. So you can train with a friend or relative and split the cost. Whatever the cost is you are worth it if you need the extra guidance. If you cut back on a few things and you might find that you really can afford a Personal Trainer. You'll life is far more valuable to you than some of the frivolous things that we buy. Examine your needs and see if this step is the right one for you.

SET UP A GYM

AREA IN YOUR HOME

This lesson is for all categories previously listed. If you are able to get a gym membership or even if you just want to pay to take fitness classes you will need to set up an area in your home for a at home workout. There will be many occasions where things come up. Life throws curve balls at times, so we have to be prepared. Just this winter the south had a terrible unusual snowstorm. If you know anything about the south and snow then you will know that we were at a standstill for days. If I had not had my small area set up for a quick at home workout I would have had to go days without a good workout.

If the area is large or small it really does not matter. Most of the time people will just have a small piece of cardiovascular equipment in their homes to use in case they are unable to make it to the gym on occasion. So you could purchase a bike, a treadmill, a boxing bag, or even something as small as a jump rope. If you are lucky enough to have an extra room that you can turn into a make shift gym then you should do that. In a later lesson

I will give you a list of things that you can fill the room with in order to get a great workout in. Some of my best workouts have been in my make shift gym in my garage. That maybe because there is no one there to watch me so I am able to cut all the way loose.

Pump up the ─────── Activity to lose

Your results will come by working hard. Reversing all of the damage that we have done to ourselves does not come by osmosis. The pounds will not magically disappear. In order for your body to show changes you must change some if not all of your behavior. If you are out for your morning walk you might want to get your upper body involved by adding in a little fist pumping action. Our bodies are used to walking so where is the challenge in that? In order to see the real change that you desire you have to work hard for it. Do things that will challenge your body and get your heart rate up. If you have been checked and cleared by the doctor it probably won't kill you. Our bodies were made to do this so it will soon adjust to the recent stresses that you have placed upon it. Once it does then it will come a time to change it up and challenge it with new things.

LEAVE THE CHATTER FOR LATER

When you are working out, Work out! Nothing irritates me more than to come into the gym and run into the chatter boxes. No, I am not anti-social, but my gym time is just that, my gym time. I train myself about 4am Monday thru Friday so it is hard enough for me to get out of bed at that hour to get to the gym. The last thing that I want to do is chatter. It defeats the purpose of going if all you are going to do is stand around and talk. If you have a workout partner and you feel it is becoming more of a therapy session, then reevaluate whether you should try it solo or try and find a less talkative person to train with. The same thing goes for the cell phone and chatter. Your workouts should only be an hour or so. If you can go without speaking on the phone for that long please do. Try to devote that one hour or so just for you with no conversation distraction. You'll find if you leave the chatter for later you will work harder.

BUY YOURSELF A NEW WORKOUT OUTFIT

Nothing will make you feel better than looking great in a new workout outfit. Having something nice to workout in is no different than wearing your favorite suit. You feel like a million bucks while you are wearing it. My philosophy is that when you look good you feel good.

Those two things go together always. Whether you workout at home or at the gym having a nice new outfit especially after you have reach a few of your short term goals will have you to see yourself in a different light. If you are a gym member, try to look nice every time you go. Not for anyone else, but for yourself. If you look presentable you will not focus on your short comings. Your mind will accentuate your best features. That alone will push you to train harder.

ESSENTIAL GYM EQUIPMENT THAT MAKE YOUR LIFE EASIER

We all cannot afford or make time to go to the gym and even if we can in earlier lessons I explained that there will be times that you cannot make it there. It is probably a great idea to have a few items at home if you are unable to attend a gym. There are many, many items but here is a good short list of things that helped me with my in home clients as well as my training. I hope it will be beneficial for you as well.

1. *One piece of cardio equipment: I.e.: Treadmill, bike, ECT. I have a potable boxing bag that I use in my home. Of course you will need to have a pair of boxing gloves and sand to go with this item. This is quick and burns lots of calories.*

2. *Resistance bands: I love these because I travel a lot. They take up nearly no space and come in different resistant strengths from extra light-super heavy.*

3. *Medicine ball: This is a handy tool that can work any part of your body. Most people associate it with abdominal work. These balls come in different weight sizes and will challenge your entire body.*

4. *Hand weights: Hand weights are one that most people are familiar with. They come in different weight sizes from 1lb all the way up to several hundred. You can work your entire body with hand weights. Using them will help you burn more calories than if you use the stationary machines because you are supporting yourself.*

5. *Jump rope: they take up little or no space and are portable for travel. Jumping rope burns mega amounts of calories. If you do not have a jump rope mock jump roping will work great as well.*

6. *Hula hoop: A hula hoop is not only a calorie burner but it is fun. It is almost not a workout at all because it will take you back to your youth.*

7. *Kettle bells: If you are more advanced and have been trained to use a kettle bell this is a great way to burn fat and build lean muscle.*

HELPFUL THINGS TO

HAVE WHEN YOU ARE

GOING TO THE GYM

There are a few essential to have when you are traveling to the gym. Here is a list of things that helped me along the way and that almost every gym goers has or should have.

1. *Water Bottle: It is essential for you to have a water bottle while working out. We lose water through sweat and it is very important that we put it back in through our water intake. This will also help you keep track of how much you are drinking.*

2. *A towel: A lot of gyms do not have towels for you to use so you might as well get into the habit of bringing your own. This will help to keep you dry and for you to put over the equipment as you use it.*

3. *Fitness journal: We spoke earlier about the importance of having a workout log. This will track your progress by keeping track of what exercise you are doing , how much weight you are lifting, and how many times. You want to bring it with you and write in it every time you workout. When the workload that you are doing gets easier then you can bump it up 5lbs or so.*

4. *Gym bag: Invest in a good bag and one that you love. Get in the habit of packing it before hand so it is ready to go. If lockers are available at your facility, don't forget your lock to lock it up.*

5. *Music Player: I don't train if I don't have my music player. Like I stated earlier the songs that I have chosen pushes me to do my best. I put my headphones on and I am in the zone.*

No more excuses

This lesson is a hard one that will probably apply to all of us at some point on our journey. There are so many excuses that we can come up with not to workout. We will say things such as I'm too tired, I overslept, it's too cold, it's too hot, and the list goes on forever. The bottom line is that is all they are is excuses. If you or someone in your family is not dead or maimed then it is imperative that you make some time to exercise. Exercise is such an important entity in your world. It helps to combat against so many aliments and diseases. You do not have to work out for hours on end to make a difference. You do not have to be a star athlete, a body builder or already in shape to workout but you need to stop making excuses for not starting, or intermitting your fitness. Let's get up and have no more excuses.

Stop spinning your wheels

Starting and stopping your fitness plan is one sure way to start spinning your wheels. What I mean by spinning your wheels is you are hot and cold. You will do great with your new lifestyle for about a month and then something out of the ordinary happens and you fall off and stay off for about two months. This then becomes a pattern in your life, starting for a month and stopping for two or three months. This behavior pattern is not good at all. No one has to be perfect at this but your good days must outweigh your bad days. It goes back to earlier lessons by having to change some things in your life. For me, I notice that when I hang out late with friends that alone throws me off of my routine and schedule for probably a couple of days , but when I was new at this I would be off for about a month. So, I limit my late nights in order to avoid the falling off. If you do not modify some of your life your body won't change and you will just spin your wheels. Who wants to do that? Who wants to go and workout only to maintain what they have. That is fine if you are at your goal but when you are not, it makes getting up in the morning at 5 or 6 a.m. without results very difficult for you and hard to understand. This will prove to be very disappointing and discouraging. In the end it might cause you to quit all together.

In order to not spin you wheels, here are a few small & easy tips that helped me see great results:

1. *You will have to modify your lifestyles and habits. If you are finding that you are missing scheduled workouts because of habits you have, you might need to move that habit to a day that you do not train or cut it out altogether.*

2. *Chose your workout times carefully. If you are not a morning person it would be very unwise to set up a time for you to train in the morning. Remember, baby steps you will get there one day.*

3. *Control your eating. You don't know how many times I have see people kill themselves at the gym for hours and later on you see them at the fast food restaurants ordering the entire menu. That is a prime example of spinning your wheels. They look the same year after year and not being able to control their eating is the reason why.*

4. *Look at this as just what it is a lifestyle change. People go on and off diets, they eventually end, but a lifestyle is a change you make for the long haul. Remember that it is a marathon, not a sprint.*

Trust me it is not all about the way you look. It is

mostly about your numbers at your physician's office. First and foremost you want those numbers to improve. Let's face it they are what keep you with life and having it more abundantly. The way you look doesn't count if you are ailing or dead. Looking great is just an added bonus. Keeping your focus and reminding yourself of your goals will help you not to spin your wheels. When your wheels start moving ahead you see progress.

LIST OF MY MOTIVATIONAL SONGS

I love music and I am rarely without a music player in my ear. Maybe I am biased when I say that music is partially responsible for a lot of my transformation. These are some songs that have pushed me to go passes my limits. These songs spoke to me in some form or fashion. Some of the songs are thought provoking and some just made me move. Some of them are old and some are current. The actually list is much, much longer than the book would allow, but these are just a few of my favorites. I hope you make your own list and you are welcome to chose from my top 50. Enjoy.

1. *Lose Yourself-Eminem*
2. *I believe- Fantasia*
3. *Stronger- Kanye West*
4. *Bleed it out- Linkin Park*
5. *Hate on me- Jill Scott*

6. *Push it to the limit- Rick Ross*

7. *Survivor- Destiny's Child*

8. *Just Fine- Mary J. Blige*

9. *Golden – Jill Scott*

10. *Imma be-The Black Eyed Peas*

11. *Perfect- Pink*

12. *My Sacrifice- Creed*

13. *Back Then- Mike Jones*

14. *Till I collapse- Eminem &Nate Dogg*

15. *Bodies- Drowning **Pool***

16. *Hello, Good Morning- Diddy*

17. *Rock Star- Nickelback*

18. *Through the Wire- Kanye West*

19. *Break the walls down- Jim Johnston*

20. *20 Feet Tall Eyrakah Badu*

21. *Imagine Me- Kirk Franklin*

22. *All eyes on me- Tupac*

23. *H.A.M.- Kayne West & Jay Z*

24. *Hustle Hard- Ace Hood*

25. *The Best In Me- Marvin Sapp*

26. *Move your Body- Nina Skyy*

27. *Maria, Maria- Carlos Santana*

28. *No Hands- Waka Flocka Flame*

29. *Turnin Me On- Nina Skyy & Baby Cham*

30. *I'm Me- Lil Wayne*

31. *Last Chance- Ginuwine*

32. *Mistreated- Shawn Kane*

33. *f*** you- Ceelo Green*

34. *Fighter- Christina Aguilera*

35. *Welcome to the jungle- Gun & Roses*

36. *I need you now- Smokie Norfolk*
37. *Hustle & Flow (It aint over for me)- Terrence Howard*
38. *Big Girls don't cry- Fergie*
39. *Rolling in the deep- Adele*
40. *N★★★★★ in Paris- Kanye West & Jay Z*
41. *Bad Girl- Usher*
42. *This is why I'm Hot- Mims*
43. *Get Me Bodied- Beyonce*
44. *So Fresh, so clean- Outcast*
45. *Whip my hair- Willow*
46. *Stronger- Kelly Clarkson*
47. *Living on a prayer- Bon Jovi*
48. *Miss Independent- Ne-Yo*
49. *Closer- Goapele*
50. *Brighter Day – Kirk Franklin*

More Random Tips

1. *Don't spend your whole day working out thinking that it will help you to lose the weight faster because it won't. It will only make you loathe it and could possibly lead to injury or burnout.*

2. *Staying in the sauna is not a workout. So many people skip the workout to spend 30-40 minutes in the hot sauna thinking that they can sweat away the pounds magically. You will lose water but as soon as you drink something guess what its back. So use that time for working out. The results will come out better for you.*

3. *Push yourself. I'll admit it is hard. No one that I know loves to workout. Most people who workout just love the results that it gives. So stop making excuses for not exercising.*

4. *Remember Rome was not built in a day and neither will you. When you look at pictures of people with beautiful physiques that inspire you, keep in mind that it took time for them to look like that. They*

constantly kept chipping away at their mountain and the beautiful picture is the result. If you stick with it someone will look at your picture one day and be inspired.

5. Don't give up on your entire journey for one day of failure. If you had a horrible day so what? Tomorrow is a brand new day and you are allowed to start again.

6. If you are weight training try doing that first followed by your cardio. Weight training requires proper form and technique so perform it while you are fresh to maintain both.

7. Changing your mind changes your body. The moment your mindset changes, then the body will follow.

8. Ladies do not be afraid of lifting weights. It will not make you bulky or "too big". It will burn more fat and give you long lean muscle.

Basic Workout Definitions

1. **Cardiovascular Training**- *A cardiovascular workout is one that is focused on increasing your heart rate to burn fat and strengthens your heart. This will commonly be referred to as cardio.*

2. **Weight Training**-*System of conditioning involving lifting weights, especially for strength*

and endurance. This can also be called strength training.

3. **Rep-** *One execution of any exercise*
4. **Set-** *A combination of any number of reps of one exercise*
5. **Workout-** *The routine, Specific exercises weights, sets, and reps for one or more body parts.*
6. **Intensity-** *The degree in which the body worked in the particular exercise*
7. **Aerobic-** *Activity that uses mainly oxygen to burn fuel at low to moderate levels of intensity.*
8. **Anaerobic-** *Activity that uses mainly the body's stored fuel for its energy. Weight training is an example of an anaerobic activity.*
9. **Dumbbell-** *small weight you can hold in each hand*
10. **Free weights-** *The round shaped weighted plates that are used on barbells and weight racks*

These are a few definitions that you will more than likely hear throughout your Fitness journey. Familiarize yourself with the basic language.

Recipes

I am definitely not a chef, but I know what I like. As I gained more and more knowledge on what our bodies need to get healthy and fit I began to play with flavors and different foods. Trust me there were a lot of trial and error situations where a whole lot of dishes just did not make it, but here are a few of my favorites that continue to help me through my journey. I'm sure you will eventually have some of your own. I hope that you enjoy!

Protein coffee (a great pick me up for coffee lovers)

1-2 scoops of vanilla or chocolate protein

6-8 cubes of ice

1-2 packages of stevia sweetener

6-8 oz of flavored black coffee

½ cup-1cup of unsweetened almond milk

Take all of these ingredients and mix them in a blender or shaker. Enjoy 1 **serving**

Chicken salad

1-2 oz. of cooked, skinless chicken breast

2-3 chopped celery sticks

¼ cup of chopped onions

1tablespoon of plain Greek yogurt

1oz of walnuts

¼ cup of raisins

¼ teaspoon of sea salt

¼ teaspoon of pepper

Mix all ingredients, refrigerate and serve chilled

2-3 servings

Yogurt parfait

1 cup of Greek yogurt

1oz. of frozen, sliced strawberries

1oz. of frozen blueberries

1oz. frozen blackberries or raspberries

1oz. of almonds

1 package of stevia

Layer ingredients and refrigerate overnight

1 serving

Yogurt muesli

1cup of Greek yogurt

½ cup of muesli

1 package of stevia

10-15 blueberries

Mix ingredients and refrigerate overnight **1 serving**

Lean turkey wraps

1lb cooked, extra lean turkey seasoned as desired

4-6 iceberg lettuce leaves

½ cup of low fat or veggie cheese

½ cup of salsa

Spoon turkey into the middle of lettuce leaves

Add ½ tablespoon of salsa

Sprinkle cheese on turkey

Fold lettuce

Hold together with a toothpick

Serve chilled or after preparation

Makes 7-8 servings

All Essential Sandwich

2 slices of Ezekiel bread

1 thinly sliced chicken breast

3-4 cucumber slices
A few spinach leaves
1 slice of low fat or veggie cheese
1 teaspoon of hummus
Arrange sandwich as desired. This sandwich can also be placed on a Panini maker for about a minute to provide a better hold. **1 serving**

Protein pancakes

1cup of whole grained rolled oats
1 scoop of vanilla protein powder
3-4 egg whites
A dash of cinnamon
Mix ingredients
Spray pan lightly with olive oil spray
Heat pan on low heat setting for about 1 minute
Pour mixture onto the pan
Cook until brown on both sides
Makes 3-4 servings

Homemade vegetable soup

1 whole sliced carrot
2-3 chopped green onions
1 sliced zucchini
1 sliced yellow squash
¼ cup of white onion (diced)
¼ cup of spinach leaves
2 cups of low sodium chicken broth
1 cup of purified water
1/3 teaspoon of sea salt

¼ teaspoon of pepper

Mix broth, water, salt, and pepper in a pot

Cook carrot, zucchini, squash, and white onions in broth and water until tender

Simmer for 15 minutes

Add spinach and green onions

Continue simmering for another five minutes

Makes3-4 servings

Fruit Smoothie

8-10 Blueberries (fresh or frozen)

5-10 sliced strawberries (Fresh or Frozen)

1 small frozen Banana

8-10 Blackberries (Fresh or frozen)

3-4 cubes of ice

½ cup of freshly juiced apple or pear

Handful of spinach leaves

¼ cup of unsweetened almond milk

Add all ingredients in a blender and blend until smooth

Makes 2-4 servings

Veggie Drink

1 Carrot

½ apples

½ small beet peeled

Handful of spinach

1-2 celery sticks

¼ cucumbers

3-4 cubes of ice

4-6 oz of purified water

Place ingredients into blender and blend until smooth
Makes 2 servings

<u>Nut Medley</u>
1 oz almonds
1 oz walnuts
1 oz pecans
1 tbs of honey
1 tsp of cinnamon

Mix all ingredients together in a bowl until fully mixed
Broil in oven for about 2-5 minutes or until desired
crispiness
Makes 1-2 servings

<u>Protein Muffins</u>
1 cup of muesli
1 whole egg
2 egg whites
1/3 cup of almond milk
¼ tbs of cinnamon
2 packages of stevia
1 tbs of honey
1 tbs of almond butter
1tsp of pure vanilla extract
1/3 cup of flaxseed meal
1 scoop of vanilla or chocolate protein

Mix all ingredients together in bowl

Spray a small 12 or 24 muffin pan lightly with olive oil spray

Spoon mixture into pan

Cook on 400 degrees for 12-15 minutes or until toothpick comes out clean.

Makes 10-12 servings

Stuffed Bell pepper

4 Medium green peppers

1 lb of lean or very ground lean ground turkey (cooked)

¼ cup of onions (finely chopped)

½ cup of Quinoa (cooked)

½ red tomatoes (diced)

½ cup of low fat mozzarella cheese

Neatly cut tops off of peppers and set to the side

Clean out the insides of peppers

Mix all the ingredients except cheese in a medium sized bowl

Divide mixture up and spoon into peppers being careful not to fill too high

Sprinkle a little cheese on top and place pepper tops back on

Cooking twine can be used to hold pepper together

Bake in oven on 350 degrees for 20-25 minutes

Makes 4 servings

Baked Kale

10-12 kale leaves

¼ tsp of sea salt

Olive oil spray

Arrange kale leaves on a foiled lined pan. Spray lightly
bottom of pan with olive oil spray

Lay the leaves flat lightly spry the top

Sprinkle sea salt on leaves sparingly

Bake in oven on 400 degrees for about 10-15 minutes
or until crispy

1-2 servings

This is a great potato chip substitute snack

Rice Cake Delight

1 unsalted rice cake

1 tsp of hummus

4-6 thinly sliced cucumbers

2-3 thinly sliced tomatoes

Spread hummus on rice cake

Arrange cucumber and tomato slices on top

1 serving

Curry Tuna

1 Can of Albacore tuna in water

2 medium celery sticks (diced)

2 tbs of Greek yogurt

¼ tsp of curry powder

Mix ingredients together in a bowl & refrigerate
Serve chilled
About 2-3 servings

Baked apple slices
1 Granny Smith Apple
1 tbs of honey
¼ tsp of cinnamon

Mix ingredients in bowl
Bake in oven on 350 degrees for 10-12 minutes or until
apple is tender

1 serving

Cottage cheese snack
1 cup of cottage cheese
1 tsp of natural peanut butter or almond butter
10-12 unsweetened raisins
Mix together and serve
1 serving

Sweet Potato Surprise

1 small sweet potato
1 cored and peeled apple (boiled until soft)
1 tsp of honey
1 tsp of pumpkin pie spice 1/3 cup of raisins

1/3 cup of almond milk

Blend ingredients until smooth and serve

Makes 1-2 servings

Banana Dessert

1 soften banana

¼ tsp of cinnamon

1 scoop of vanilla protein powder

½ cup of almond milk

Mash banana until smooth

Blend all ingredients together and refrigerate until chilled

1-2 servings

Mini pizza

1 Ezekiel bread muffin

2 oz of cooked lean turkey

1/4 cup of onions

6-8 black olives

1 jalapeño pepper sliced

2 sliced grape tomato

1/3 cup of mozzarella cheese

10 spinach leaves

2 tsp of organic tomato paste

Spread tomato paste on each half of muffin

Arrange ingredients in order that you desire leaving cheese to sprinkle on top last

Bake in oven on 30 degrees for 10-12 minutes or until cheese is melted

2 servings
Other ingredients can be added or subtracted to better suit your taste

Egg white vegetable omelet

2-3 egg whites
¼ cup of onion (finely chopped)
1/3 cup of green peppers (diced)
1/3 cup red peppers (diced)
½ tomato (diced)
10-15 spinach leaves
1/4 veggie cheese

Sauté onions, red peppers and green peppers, in lightly olive oil sprayed pan and set aside
Cook egg whites in a lightly sprayed olive oil pan
When half way done cooking add in cooked pepper onion mixture on one side of omelet
Add spinach and cheese and fold over
Cook until fully cooked flipping several times if necessary

1-2 servings

Salmon Skews

1-2 oz of salmon
1 zucchini sliced

1 squash sliced
½ white onion
Olive oil spray
Arrange ingredients on skew in random order
Spray all sides lightly with olive oil spray
Place on foiled pan
Bake in oven on 400 degrees for 15-20 minutes or until
salmon is completely cooked and vegetables are tender
Makes about 6 skews (3 servings)
**Other vegetables and chicken breast can also be
used in place of salmon to suit your taste**

Lean Turkey Spaghetti
1 lb of lean or extra lean ground turkey
½ cup of chopped onions
½ cup of green peppers (chopped)
1 cup of tomatoes (diced)
1 package of quinoa pasta

Sautee onions and green peppers in a small amount of
light olive oil and set aside
Cook ground turkey on stove top until fully cooked
Follow listed directions cooking quinoa pasta

Mix sautéed green peppers, onions, diced tomatoes and
cooked ground turkey and place on top of quinoa pasta
Makes about 8-10 servings

Lean bison patties
1 package of bison or buffalo meat

¼ cup of chopped onions

1 tbs of curry powder

1 tsp of sea salt

1 tsp of ground pepper

1 whole egg

2 egg whites

1/3 of flaxseed meal

Place all ingredients in a large bowl

Mix thoroughly

Roll out flat golf sized ball meatballs

Place in oven on 350 degrees for 25–30 minutes or until meat is fully cooked

Ground lean turkey or very lean beef can also be used for this recipe

Makes 6-8 small patties

About 4 servings

There are many exercises that will get you going in the right direction. I came up with a list of my top ten; anyone who has been cleared by their physician can perform these. These exercises can be done anywhere, at home, on vacation, at work on a break, so there are no excuses for not doing them. They do not require any equipment (but you are welcome to add weight when this becomes too easy). Your body will let you know when this happens. These exercises are using your bodyweight only. They will help you get used to getting up and getting moving. Consistently try a few out at a time until you build up your strength and tolerance levels in a few weeks. Later on try performing the whole list. With practice and being true consistency, you will be able to repeat the set of exercises 2-3 times. Great luck to you and let's get busy!!!

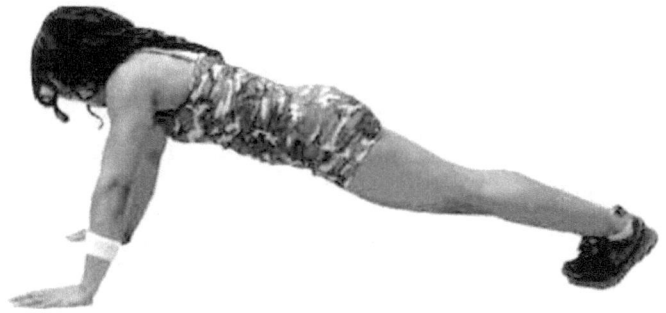

Pushups are a great exercise to build upper body strength and endurance. They can be done as pictured or with bent knees. They are to be performed with a straight back in lined with your spine, chest up, pushing down

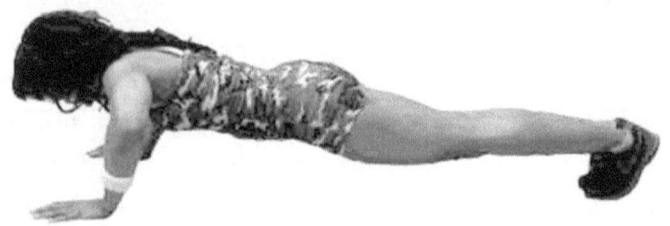

bending at the elbows and back up again.

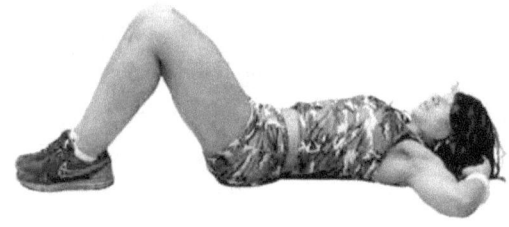

Crunches are great for strengthening the abdominal region keeping in mind that you still must keep a close eye on your nutrition and cardio in order to see your hard word. The start position is flat on the floor with no arch in your back with your legs bent at a 90 degree angle. Inhale as you go up as far as you can hold for a second or two and blow the breath at the top. After which you come back down to the start position.

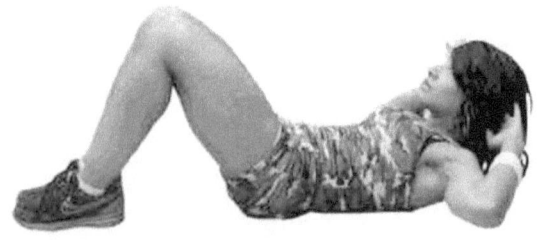

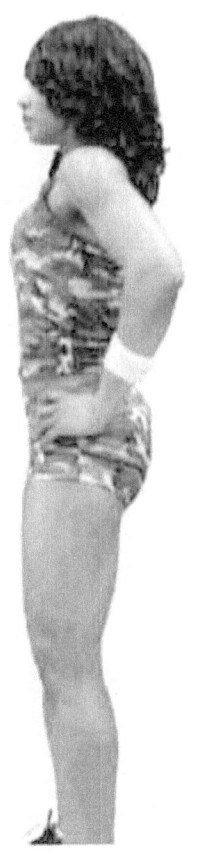

Squats are one of my favorite exercises. Working the big muscles such as legs will help to burn many calories. You will start with your feet about should width apart leaving them flat on the ground. Bring your body down as if you were going to sit in a chair and hold that for about 2 seconds and then return to the start squeezing back to the top. Be careful not to let you knees overlap your toes and remember to keep your heels down.

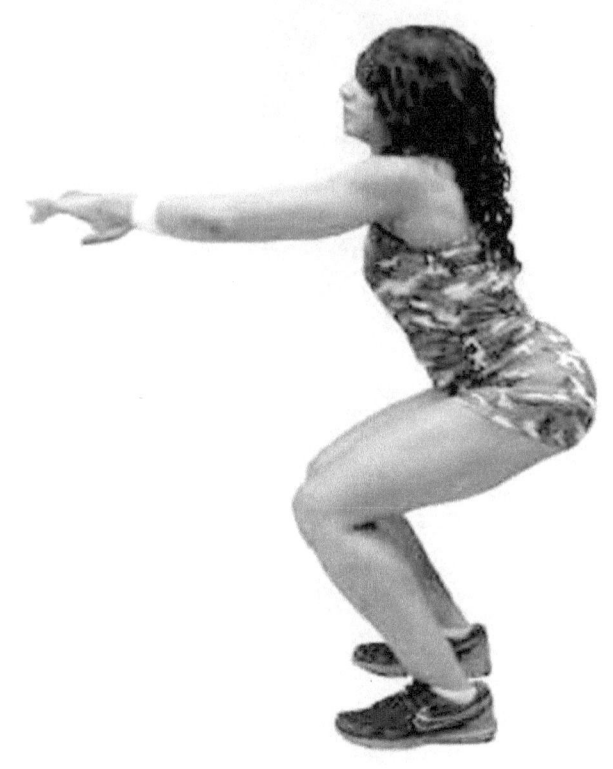

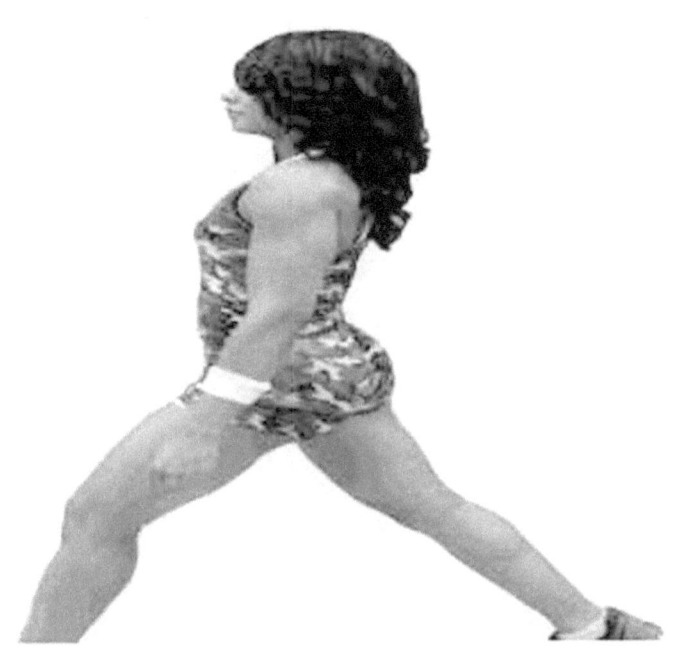

Lunges are a girl's best friend. They help build and strengthen your legs as well as your gluteus (Buttocks). Stand with legs in a split position with the back legs heel up, keeping your torso erect, drop down and hold for a couple of seconds. You would then squeeze it back up to the top. You could alternate or do one leg at a time. Do not let your knee go over your toe.

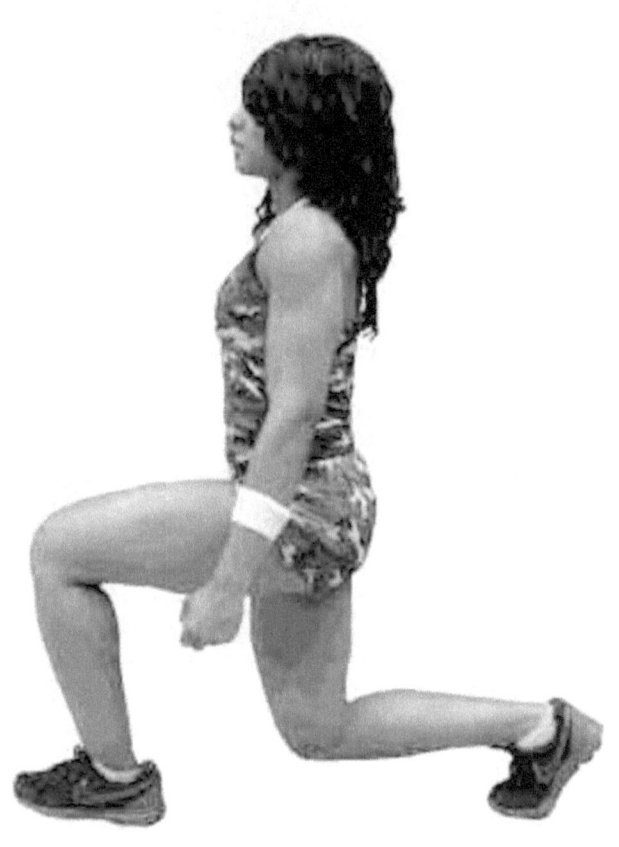

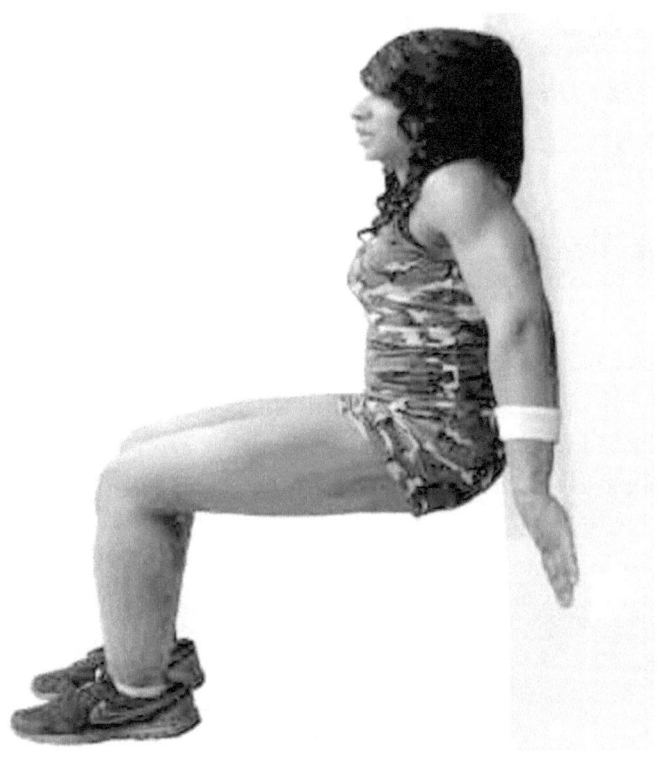

Wall sits help to strengthen your legs while building endurance. Find a wall and sit pretending there is a chair underneath you. Your head and hands are flat against the wall. You will hold that position anywhere from 15 seconds to one minute. Keep in mind that you might not be able to go all of the way down at first but you will get there with practice and patience I promise. As you advance weight can also be added if desired.

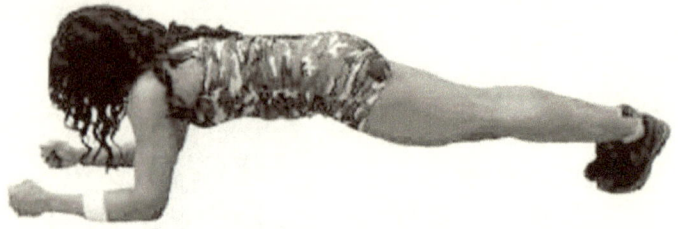

The plank is a great core exercise. You will feel this exercise in several places on your body. As demonstrated lie on the floor getting up on your forearms. You will keep your back straight and flat keeping your buttocks out of the air. Hold in this position anywhere from 15 seconds to 2 minutes. Advance the time as you get stronger. Weight can also be added to this exercise as you advance as well as several variations.

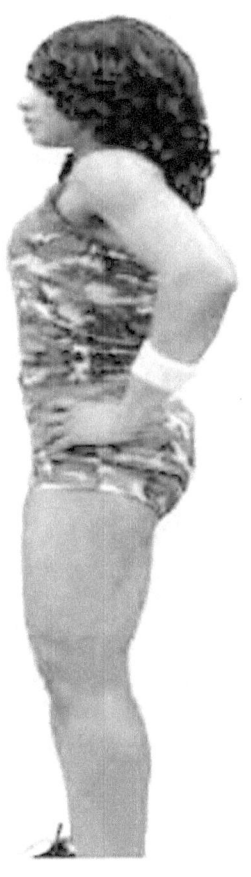

Jump squats can build muscle and be an asset to building your cardio capacity. Jump squats are performed at first like a squat but adding a jump into it landing back in a squat position. When you land make sure to land softly back on your heels and not on your toes. In the beginning you may only be able to do a few of these at a time before resting but like everything else practice makes perfect.

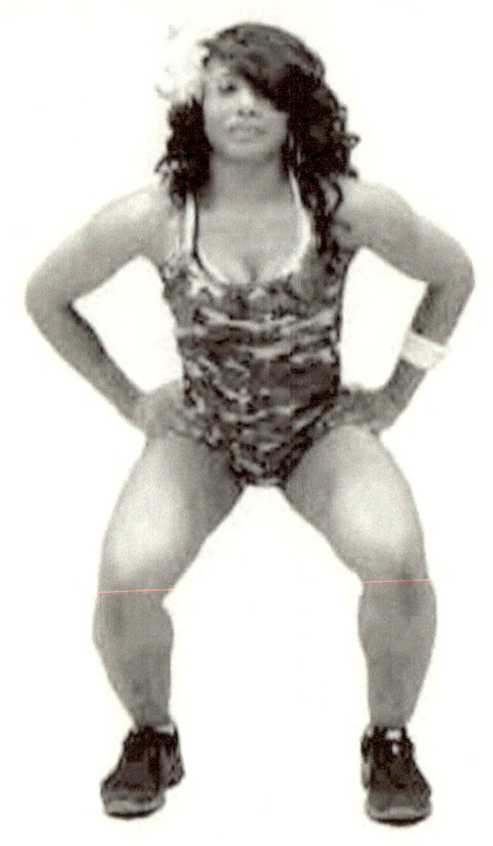

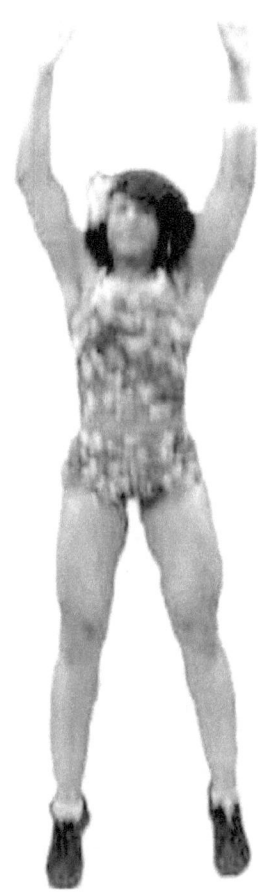

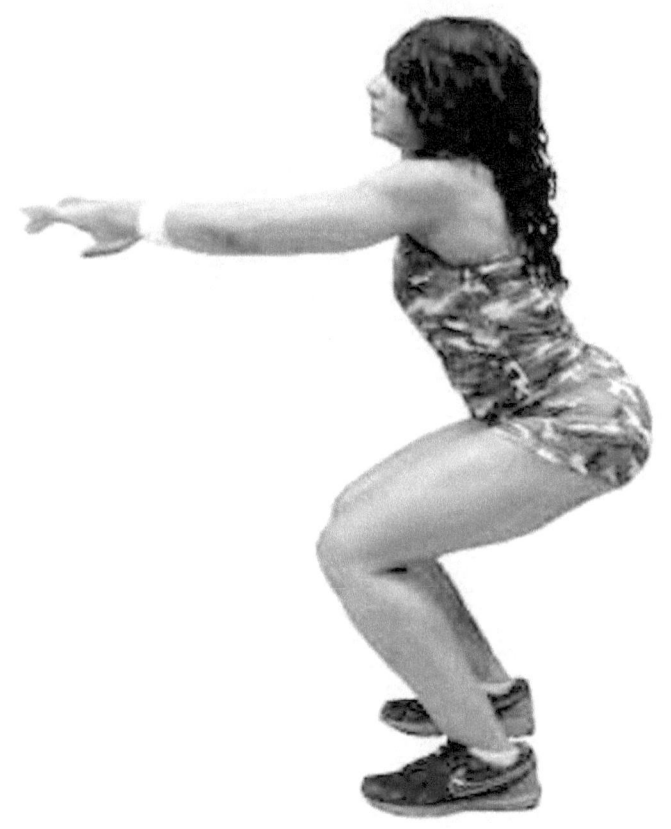

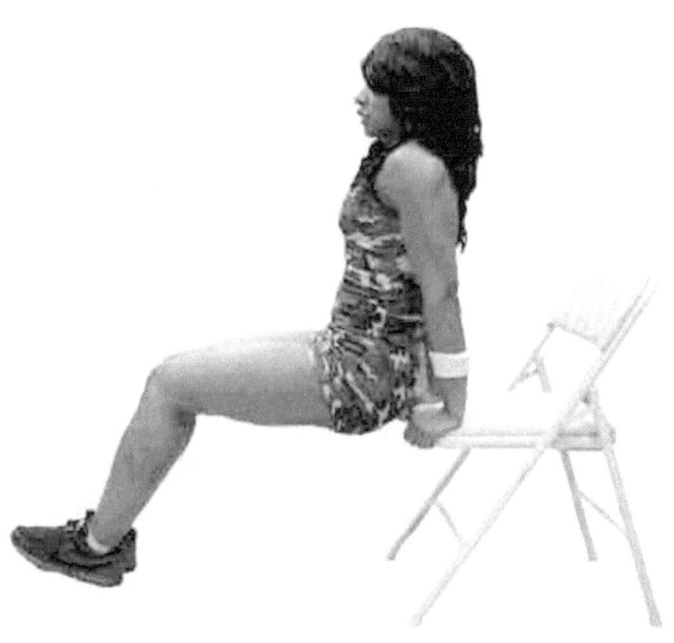

Chair dips build the triceps (the back of the arm).
Find a sturdy chair or a bench, sit on the chair and slowly
slide yourself out to the edge of the chair. Slowly bend

your elbows about 90 degrees and hold for 1-2 seconds before returning back to the starting position.

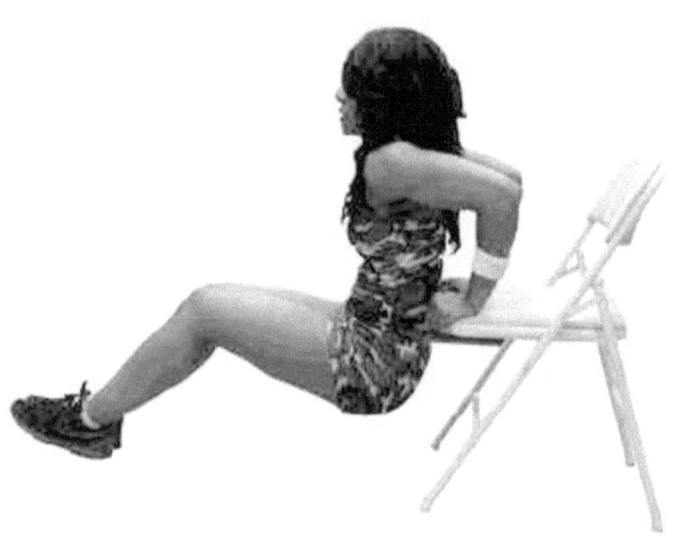

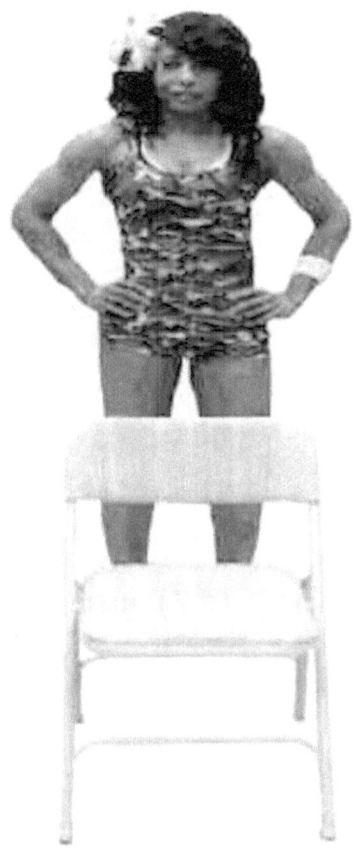

Leg swings help to build the legs, cardiovascular system, endurance coordination and balance. Make sure you find an object that you are able to get your leg all of the way over. You might have to begin with a kids chair or a small step stool. Stand behind the chair or object without swaying your back swing your leg over to the other side alternating or completing one side at a time.

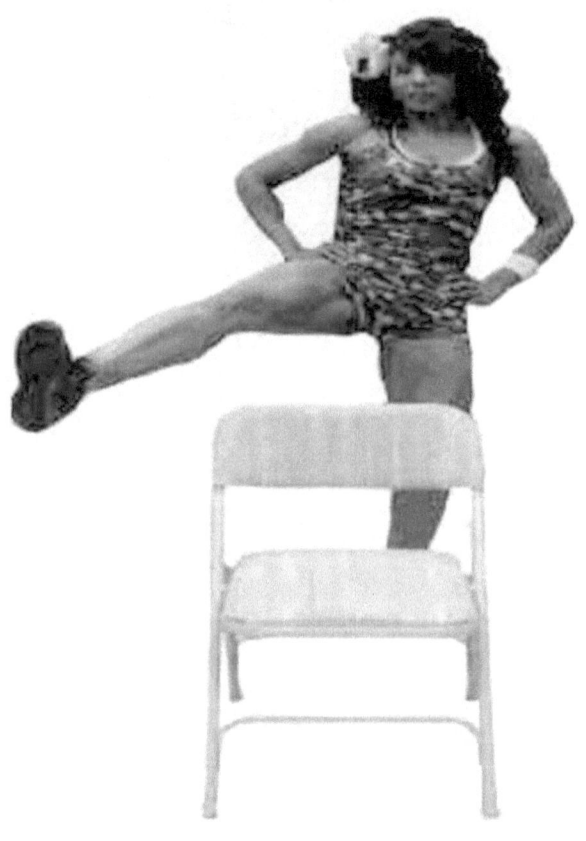

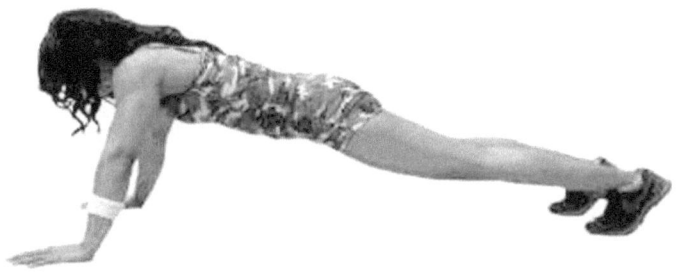

Mountain Climbers work on building cardio as well as strength gaining in the entire body. Get up in the pushup position and alternate each leg bringing it up to chest level. Perform this exercise for about 20 seconds to two minutes adding time as you get more advanced.

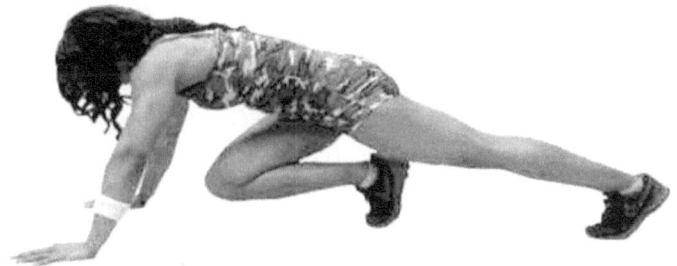

ACKNOWLEDGEMENTS

Thank you God! My main purpose on this earth is to serve you. What better way to do it than by serving your people. Father there are many who are hurting and dying from lack of knowledge. I thank you God for giving me the mind to want to reach out and help. I thank you Lord, for healing me spiritually, physically and mentally. Without you Lord I am nothing and all that I am I owe to you. *" But I discipline my body and bring it into subjection, lest, when I have preached to others, I myself should become disqualified"* 1 Corinthians 9:27

I thank my supportive husband Chris Jefferies. Thank you for believing in my dreams even when I didn't.

I thank my family for all of their love and support. My parents Mr. & Mrs. Eddie & Diane Waters. I thank my sisters Rena Muldrow, Kim Langford, & Tara Brown. I Love you guys always.

I want to thank my small, close circle of friends for listening when I need to talk. I love you all like family. In no particular order, Connie, D'Juan, Cherice , Erica, Teresa , Kendra, Will, Darrall , Constance , Lawrence , Adrian , John, Reggie, Gabby, Camille, Kevin & King. No last names because you all know who you are!!! I have talked all of your ears off about my life, hopes and dreams Thank you for listening when I was going through!

Notes from Alura

I want to help heal the world. Is that too tall of an order to take on? I don't think it is. I love my fellow man so I just want to do my part to help to educate and eventually heal others. This is a life long journey in which I will be the first to admit isn't all of the time easy to stick with but it is necessary and worth every bit of effort that we put into it. Everything about this lifestyle is a challenge, but was it suppose to be? If we ourselves make a change by introducing great eating habits and exercise into our lives we can then teach our kids those changes they will then teach their children and so on and so forth. And that is how we will win and reclaim our bodies and lives back. It just has to start from somewhere and from somebody. God knows the last 15 months have been almost a living hell on earth for me. I should be 400lbs right now just by eating all of the foods that I would have normally eaten to sooth my pain. But I chose a different route this time. It started out as just a distraction and ended up as a great journey for me. This is a journey that I am still on and one that I plan to be on until the day that I die. My sacrifices are making me better. I'm being healed from the inside out and I love it. I want to share this with all who will listen saying that we no longer have to have sickness in our bodies and minds brought on by the wrong kinds of foods and lack of activity. Armed with knowledge we can take our power back. We will no longer listen to profit makers on what is good for us. We will have the education ourselves to decide for what's best on our behalf. (I know there are many that don't believe)But the word of God says, *"My people are lost for lack of knowledge"* and that is what we need in order to move forward. The bible also states that *"Whatever you eat or drink or whatever you do, you must do all for the glory of God". Whether you believe in God or not most believe that our bodies are our temple so therefore we must take care of it. God made us stewards over our bodies we must choose to be a good one.* The bottom line is that it comes down to sacrifice, and who better to sacrifice for than yourself? I'm hoping that *today is Your Monday* to do something about you situation because I know that you can make it out. Start today, whatever day it might be. Peace & Blessings

www.ingramcontent.com/pod-product-compliance
Lightning Source LLC
Chambersburg PA
CBHW051444280526
45785CB00003B/1423